The FOOD TRAP

Breaking Its Hidden Control

PAMELA M. SMITH, R.D.

Creation House
Lake Mary, Florida

Creation House
Strang Communications Company
600 Rinehart Road
Lake Mary, FL 32746
(407) 333-0600

Unless otherwise noted, all Scripture quotations are taken from
the Holy Bible, New International Version. Copyright © 1973,
1978, 1984, International Bible Society. Used by permission.

The Twelve Steps are reprinted with permission of Alcoholics
Anonymous World Services Inc. Permission to reprint the
Twelve Steps does not mean that AA has reviewed or approved
the contents of this publication nor that AA agrees with the
views expressed herein. AA is a program of recovery from alcoholism. Use of the Twelve Steps in connection with programs
and activities which are patterned after AA but which address
other problems does not imply otherwise.

Second printing, November 1990
Third printing, May 1991
Fourth printing, August 1991
Fifth printing, October 1992
Sixth printing, March 1994
Seventh printing, June 1994

The FOOD TRAP

ACKNOWLEDGMENTS

With utmost appreciation to my husband, Larry, for his consistent love and support; to my daughters, Danielle and Nicole, for keeping me ever focused on my priorities in life; to my mom, who never hesitates to help and never ceases to care; to Carolyn Coats, my trusted friend, my partner in writing, who is God's very special gift to me; to David Loveless, my pastor and teacher at Discovery Church, who has provided me with a perspective of freedom that has changed my life.

CONTENTS

IS THE REFRIGERATOR LIGHT THE LIGHT OF YOUR LIFE?

- Do you make promises to *try* to control your eating but break those promises again and again?

- Do you spend a great deal of time thinking about what you have eaten or what you will be eating? Are you forever battling your feelings about food?

- Are you constantly dieting or discussing food and weight loss?

- Are you driven by a desire to be thin, equating thinness with success and being in control? Do you think about life in terms of "if only" ("if only I were thinner, then I would be married...have more friends")?

- Do you deny the physical damage or complications caused by your eating?

- Do you eat with a frenzy when under stress?

- Do you overeat because you fear food will not be available and you'll soon be hungry?
- Do you consume huge quantities of food rapidly and often secretly? Do you dispose of the evidence because you are ashamed of what you have done?
- Do you find yourself unable to stop eating?
- Do you eat to the point of nausea or vomiting or until your stomach hurts?
- Do you sometimes feel repulsed by food?
- Do you feel "good" while binging but then become overwhelmed with feelings of guilt, remorse and self-hate when you stop eating? Do you eat more to relieve these feelings?
- Do you feel exhilarated when you can control your intake of food?
- Do you avoid social engagements that involve eating if you are on a diet?
- Do you feel deprived much of the time?
- Do you feel resentful and angry because you aren't like other people when it comes to food?
- Do others view your shape differently from the way you do?

If you answer yes to many of these questions, this book is for you. Here you'll find answers that will allow you to break free of the food trap.

Caught in the Food Trap!

"There is no way I can eat this much food; I need to lose weight, not *gain it!* You're telling me that the reason I'm overweight is that I'm not eating *enough?*" Karen Thoms had been on a diet for twenty-two years. At forty-nine she was heavier than ever, tired of battling food and tired of battling the scale. She wanted to find a way to break out of the trap she was in. But what she was hearing was more than she could fathom....

———————

"I just can't imagine why anyone would choose to live life without chocolate!" Everyone who knew Toni Sanders knew how much she loved chocolate. Her weight had climbed steadily for several years, since her only child had left home. After many diets and many failures, she knew she needed help with her eating. "But *don't* tell me to give up chocolate!" she exclaimed.

———————

"I just don't have the energy I used to have. It's hard to pull out of bed in the morning, and I have certain points in the day when I'd like to come home and take a nap! Then there are the mood swings; one minute I feel pretty good, and the next minute I feel as if I've lost my best friend. My wife thinks it's because of the junk I eat all day, so she called and made an appointment with you."

Jim Martin was a thirty-four-year-old sales representative for a computer company. "As you can see, weight is not my problem. Actually I can eat whatever I want and as much as I want, and I don't gain weight. I just don't have to worry about it. But I'm beginning to wonder if I might have something wrong with me...."

———————

"Regina comes out and tells me she's been bulimic for twenty-three years and needs help!" Rich Perkins was the dynamic pastor of an active, growing church. He and Regina had been married for eighteen years and seemed to have a wonderful, open relationship. Then one memorable day Regina hit bottom and exploded with the truth: She had a secret relationship with food and could not break out of the trap!

"My friends are all so jealous of my willpower and discipline—sticking to my healthy diet. They call me to answer all their questions about nutrition and exercise." Around friends Stan was the perfect dieter. What they didn't know was that, when alone, he binged on cookies, root beer, candy bars and cheesecake. Then he would run ten to twelve miles to "work it off."

This is a book for Karen, Toni, Jim, Regina and Stan. And it's a book for you who have spent a lifetime trying to get willpower and self-discipline concerning food, only to get guilt and shame in its place!

This is a book for you who desire (maybe obsessively) a thin and healthy body, but such a body seems to be an impossible dream. It is to help you who have tried it *all* to get weight off no matter what the cost. You've tried diets, weight loss programs, drinks, potions, pills, spas. You've fasted and you've feasted; you've exercised; you've even hired people to make you exercise, but nothing works for long. You know yourself. Have you spent a lifetime dieting but weigh more than ever before?

You may not have a weight problem. Maybe your problem has even been how to keep weight *on*. Maybe you have one of those metabolisms that can burn whatever you put in. Yet, even though fatness versus thinness isn't your battle, your health is being robbed by the foods you eat: You are overcome by stress and done in by the "near-empty" supply of energy you have. You may be sick and tired of being sick and tired, but too sick and tired to do anything about it. Maybe you've just found out your blood pressure or cholesterol is high and you are at high risk for coronary disease. You know you need to change your eating patterns; you've been given a diet, yet you keep on eating in a self-destructive way.

Have you prayed and prayed for God to take away your appetite for food, but it's still there? Have you prayed and prayed for energy, but it's not there? This book is for you! You—who feel victorious in every area of your life except your weight, your energy, your moods...your eating.

If any of this sounds familiar, take heart. You are not alone.

There's Hope

I have had a private practice of nutritional counseling for twelve years, helping clients develop a life-style of wellness. I help my patients set goals for living healthy and vital lives; we develop eating and exercise plans to attain and maintain those goals.

Some patients knock on my door because they need to lose weight. Some need only to "lean down" to a more fit shape. Some need to manage stress better. Some come desiring more energy. Some come in a very ill state, needing a nutritional plan to control the symptoms of disease.

Early in my practice I sensed that the majority of my clients needed pure and simple nutritional education. They needed to learn *what* to eat, *when* to eat it and *how to balance it* in such a way to benefit their bodies. They needed to learn how to break away from the typical American eating-style while still living a normal life-style. As they heeded this education, many patients thrived and succeeded in achieving their wellness goals—more energy or leaner bodies or controlled appetites.

But I discovered another group of people whose eating problems were *not* solved simply through education. They could counsel with me and *begin* to make changes in their eating behavior, but they could not follow through and maintain any lasting change. Their eating problems seemed to be bigger than the nutritional needs of their bodies. They had a desire to eat differently, certainly *weigh* differently, but they could not succeed in these goals.

This group of patients seemed to have a dependency on food and eating that required a type of counseling far beyond the nutritional helps I had been giving. Even after learning a new way of eating that had been successful for countless others, even after seeing a measure of success in their own lives, these people would return to their old ways. With each successive attempt they were heading into deeper disillusionment and despair, as they had no idea why their attempts to get free from food and diets weren't working.

Clients from every walk of life—top executives of major corporations, homemakers, ministers, college students, teachers, retirees—all have a similar plea: I am out of control with my eating and my health!

I want to tell you what I tell them as they work out their freedom. I want to give you a new perspective about eating and food: *why you do what you do and why you don't do what you "should" do.*

Breaking out of the food trap isn't just about what you eat. Eating habits are intricately intertwined with one's emotions and one's spiritual well-being; an overdependency on food can be the barrier between you and abundant life! If you are serious about being free from slavery to food, now is the time to start.

I've tried to collect some of the best, most helpful

information on getting free from the trappings of food and unhealthy eating habits. I've included case histories to show how my patients identified and dealt with their problems. Although I've changed names and details to protect privacy, certain parts of their stories are likely to sound familiar. Your struggles may be like theirs.

Much of what I've learned has been from working with these people and their families. But then much more has been learned as I've desperately turned to God and the Bible for answers to the problems I've faced daily. I see the church being caught up in the food trap as much as, if not more than, the world, and I see the church turning to the world for answers it cannot give.

In this book I pass on to you much of what I've gleaned about breaking free from hidden, painful controls. Many people have done it. You can, too!

I have written this book to give you hope. It is about taking care of yourself. It's about what you can do to start living better. I have written it to equip you to rise up and throw off the chains that bind you to food and overeating... to dieting...to the scale...to a life with no energy. You can attain *and maintain* freedom from the food trap forever!

PART I:

HELP ME!

ONE

OUT OF CONTROL

I'm forty-something and feel as if I've been fighting a war against my body for forty-something years. I just can't lose weight and keep it off! I think I've tried every diet created. I've swallowed pills, taken shots and eaten formulated foods and powders. I've fasted and drunk protein shakes. I've prayed and been prayed for. My parents and my husband and I have spent untold amounts of money on weight-loss programs guaranteed to work. And they do work. Actually I can lose weight quite easily—but not nearly as easily as I can gain it back!"

Katie was in my office for the first time, seeking nutritional counseling for her "weight problem." At five-foot-three she weighed 172 pounds, the highest she had ever weighed. She had started dieting in junior high, and the many diets Katie had been on since had only made her fatter. She would lose thirty pounds, only to gain back thirty-five. She would lose twenty pounds and gain back thirty.

Katie's most successful diet had prompted a loss of sixty-five pounds—down to the thinnest she had ever been. Motivated by the invitation to her twenty-year high-school reunion, she had felt beautiful when she'd walked through the door. Unfortunately, she had broken the diet that night and had continued eating the rest of the weekend. A vacation and then Christmas had followed, and she had gained the entire amount back within five months.

Katie's most recent attempt at weight loss had been with one of the popular liquid-protein fasting programs, losing forty-five pounds in eight weeks. But Thanksgiving had come, and she had broken the fast—for that one day. Three weeks later she sat across the desk from me. Looking desperate and hopeless, she had gained back nineteen pounds. She couldn't face going back on a fast; nor could she face another failure.

"The truth is," she said, "I don't know why I'm even here except that this is my last resort before getting my jaws wired. Even then I'd probably gain weight on milkshakes. Maybe I just need counseling so I can learn to be happy being fat! But I know I could never really accept looking and feeling like this.

"You know, I feel as if food is my enemy, and yet I love it. I love to eat, and I love to enjoy the foods I'm eating. I can do really well on a diet for a while, but then a birthday or a holiday comes up, and I just have to eat something 'good'! I can't imagine life without eating the foods I love."

Katie ended her story with a sigh. "I can lose weight, but I just can't keep it off. I am just so tired of failing, so tired of knowing what I should do but not doing it, so tired of being fat. I am so tired of being tired."

The Sucrets Solution

Katie's real problem was not her weight. Her weight was a symptom of a bigger problem.

I compare going on a diet to taking throat lozenges for a strep throat infection. The pain you are soothing and the redness you might be reducing are symptoms of the real problem, a dangerous infection. And the infection will continue to run rampant until it is treated properly—at the root with antibiotics.

Because so few are ready or willing to look at the root problem, food, overeating and weight have a powerful grip on our lives. Just like strep throat, it takes control until we dig out the root. What is the underlying problem? Our eating patterns and perspectives about food.

The Love-Hate Relationship

A healthy relationship with food is one of friendship, where food is regarded as the nourishment it was created to be. In an improper, love-hate relationship with food we see that it has a control over us. We love the way it tastes and makes us feel, but we hate it for what it does to our bodies and how it controls our lives. Like any unhealthy relationship it results in a roller coaster of emotions: gratification and satisfaction, guilt and remorse, being "good" only to be "bad," being "on a diet" only to be "off a diet." The obsession fills our thoughts and actions, robs us of well-being, affects our self-esteem—holds us captive.

Food can be nourishment. It can be a source of pleasure. It certainly does more than satisfy hunger.

We live in a nation of people preoccupied with food. It absorbs amazing amounts of time and productivity. It is the main focus at both celebrations and funerals. We've been taught that food "makes us feel better," and we have discovered that it does. When we feel sad or depressed, a candy bar or bag of chips can be very soothing. When we are anxious or stressed, chocolate chip cookies reduce the tension. Then many people go back to their normal way of eating once the uncomfortable feeling has passed.

Others, however, do not return to their "normal" eating patterns. The logic goes something like this: If food made me feel good yesterday, it should do the same today, and if today, then tomorrow. Food doesn't let us down, even if everything else does. We eat and overeat in answer to every emotion: If we're happy, we eat. If we're sad, we eat. If we're mad, we eat. If we're frustrated, we eat. If we're feeling out of control, we eat. If we're bored, we eat. If we're celebrating, we eat. If we're grieving, we eat. (Whew!)

Why We Overeat

We overeat to cope with the stresses and insecurities of life. Overeating is a way to weather the frustration and stresses of life. It takes away the rough edges and seems to relieve the tensions, allowing us to cope. We really need time to withdraw and get a perspective on the problems, but overeating is a quicker answer.

In the introduction I mentioned Stan, a man who had the envy of all of his friends for his rigid dieting and exercise. It was not only Stan's willpower that amazed his friends; he had an uncanny expertise in the stock market. The most successful stockbroker in his firm, he had many influential clients with large financial portfolios. His success had its drawbacks: The stress was intense and constant, though he appeared to handle it well. I say "appeared" because Stan was using food to cope with that stress and tension.

Stan could not face the stresses of his job head-on, because the main source of his stress was coming from within—his driving need for perfection. He needed everything to go according to plan, but invariably it didn't. Then he resorted to a pressure-valve that would relieve the tensions and fuel his work habits: He would binge on food. But actually those sweet binges tarnished the standard of perfection he'd set for himself. The guilt he felt created even more stress to be eaten and exercised away.

We overeat to "fill the gaps" in our lives. Food becomes a friend and companion who is always there no matter what. When we're lonely, eating seems to fill the emptiness. It can substitute for love, attention and pampering. When we're happy, it's a way to celebrate—even if we're alone. When we're working hard with seemingly little recognition or appreciation, food becomes a justly earned reward and comfort.

One of the gaps we try to fill with food is our lack of self-esteem. Abusive eating is a reinforcement of the belief of being unacceptable and inadequate. A solid majority of over-eaters has suffered a damaged sense of self-worth. Few, however, make the connection between their image of themselves and their eating problems.

Unlike the world, no matter what happens, food doesn't reject or abandon us; it can be counted on. In the introduction I mentioned Toni, a woman who had accepted motherhood with joy and a sense of challenge. She had dedicated twenty years to the raising of her daughter, Meghan. Toni did so well that her daughter felt confident enough to leave the nest. She accepted a job in another state—and moved.

Toni felt so abandoned that she began to demand appreciation from the very person who could not give it to her—Meghan. Meghan was struggling with her own emotions of breaking away and could not be a support for her mother. Since Toni was going to "an empty well," she turned to food to fill the bucket.

The satisfied feeling fills in the gaps temporarily. The more Toni ate, the more weight she gained and the more depressed she got. Unfortunately, because we use food as a comforter so often, we never get the chance to fill in the gaps permanently and healthily.

We overeat to achieve a sense of identity and control. The love-hate relationship with food can become so consuming that it becomes an integral part of the core of a person's being. The relationship is yours and yours alone to control and own. No one, nothing, can interfere. For many, this relationship—what I eat—seems to be the one and only thing in life that can be controlled. You buy the food, prepare and eat it, making you totally self-sufficient in this one aspect of life, which may be the only corner over which you feel you have power. And, after all, controlling and loving food is a lot safer than controlling and loving people! For many, the "high" of food dependency is not the actual eating of the food. It is getting to that point—being obsessed with the food, buying it, preparing to eat it.

Your obsession may not be food at all; for some, food is the barrier keeping them from their obsession to be thin. To the overeater or the undereater, thinness symbolizes power and control.

I previously mentioned Karen who had been on a diet for twenty-two years. At forty-nine she was heavier than ever, tired of battling food and the scale. She wanted to find a way to break out of the trap she was in. But Karen was not willing to give up compulsive dieting, because she did not want to give up control. As long as she could control food—her enemy—she felt she had control of her world. But the truth was, she wasn't controlling it—it was controlling her.

Every time she broke her rigid dieting, she saw herself

as a failure. When she would reach her goal weight and relax a bit, she immediately gained five pounds, which led to more restrictions and more failures. She had determined that her body was defective, and she was doomed to a life of sparse eating. I'm not sure why she ever came to see me, but I suspect it was to say she had tried everything, and no one could help her

Karen listened to me at her first appointment, but she cancelled her next one and didn't come back for three years. Seeing her then surprised me, but I understood after her first sentence: "My husband has entered a recovery program for alcohol abuse, and I think he's going to need my help to learn how to eat properly." She wanted me to construct a meal plan for her husband, Robert, and she would be sure he followed it. Although I could see this was one more control she was planning to enforce, it explained a great deal to me about her eating and dieting. She had been using compulsive dieting alternating with compulsive eating to cover up her pain and shame because of her husband's disease.

We overeat to sabotage the "perfect image." An obedient, people-pleasing child can use overeating as an acceptable way to be bad or imperfect. Food is an acceptable vice, even if becoming overweight is a risk. Great satisfaction may come from secretly sabotaging a perfect image without risking rejection from family, friends or teachers. It is a passive form of rebellion, but, like any vicious cycle, it feeds itself. The more you eat, the more guilt and shame you feel; the more shame you feel, the more you eat.

Let me return to the story of Regina Perkins, minister's wife *and* minister's daughter. Regina grew up with a rigid set of rules for "acceptable behavior" and never dreamed of breaking them. She was "Papa's precious," always wearing a smile. But Regina didn't always *feel* like smiling.

25

Sometimes she felt quite resentful of being the preacher's daughter and having to be perfect. Then she would be overwhelmed with shame for these bad feelings and found she could show how "bad" she was by binging on food; no one ever knew just how rebellious she really was. Regina's resulting weight gain enhanced her passive rebellion further; she had ruined her "perfection," but to Mommy and Daddy it really wasn't her fault. Regina never let them see her overeat; they were sure it was just a "chubby" stage she was going through.

The trap became more and more vicious, and eventually her parents sought medical evaluations for her health "problem." The more she ate, the more shame she felt; the more shame she felt, the more she ate. She finally began to make herself sick after overeating, more than likely for self-punishment, but she discovered that it served to control her weight gain. So Regina developed a secret life-style of binging and purging that followed her into her marriage to Rich—until one day, when she couldn't contain the secret shame any longer.

We overeat to deal with deep-seated feelings and emotions. Events in early life can deal such deeply wounding blows that a child cannot express or even feel the full intensity of the pain of the moment. Rather, the unhealed wound festers; food becomes a balm, dulling the pain that one eventually denies existed.

Keeping one's mind on food can keep it off issues of the heart. Many of us have grown up in families that discouraged both recognizing and expressing feelings, particularly "negative" ones, such as anger, guilt or frustration. In these families, children quickly learn which feelings get positive or negative reactions from parents. Life becomes a list of emotional *shoulds* and *should nots* ("you shouldn't feel that way"; "you should be happy with what you have"; "you shouldn't think of yourself all the time"). This leaves the impression that what is being felt is bad, wrong or unacceptable. The problem with this denial—or swallowing—of emotions is that we are humans, created to feel. Birds fly; fish swim; humans feel!

Anger is an emotion particularly susceptible to being "stuffed" with food. Binging is a "safe way" to express forbidden anger. "Stuffing food" is a way to stuff the feelings, to numb them, to shut them off.

A family rule outlawing expressions of anger (which lead to conflict) or the unwritten rule that nice people don't get angry may lead you to turn the feelings of anger onto yourself. Another scenario is not unusual: Some overeaters saw inappropriate expressions of anger in childhood and grew up swearing never to repeat the pattern. The act of overeating provides an active, physical release from pent-up anger while allowing the individual to be "nice" and avoid conflict. Rather than confronting an anger-producing situation directly, you smile on the outside, rage on the inside and eat to keep it in.

Eating to stay "Mr. Nice Guy" to the world is exactly what Jim Martin had done since childhood. Weight was not a problem for Jim's high metabolism, so overeating seemed to be the perfect way to deal with rage. This was such an established pattern that Jim ceased to recognize that he ever even felt angry. He just knew that he was tired all the time.

Jim's business was in the midst of great transition when he first came to me for counseling. His commission rate and his sales district had been changed three times in two months. He had also been passed over for a promotion. Jim was aware that he was eating excessive quantities of sweets and vaguely realized that this had increased with the stress at work. He also had difficulty reporting any set eating patterns—when did he eat what? He said his eating was based on availability and the situation he faced at the moment. He was astonished to identify those situations as ones that caused him to feel angry. As long as he could eat a cookie when he began to feel "something" on the inside, he could avoid dealing with the emotion.

As long as we are eating we do not have to deal with our emotions and pain. Overeating, rather than *feeling*, really doesn't get rid of the emotions we feel; it just "stuffs them and compacts them" into brick walls. If, every time you feel angry at someone, you turn to food, you never get a chance to process and deal with that anger. Instead you've compacted it. When something occurs that releases some painful memory of your past and you turn to food, you never have an opportunity to process and release that pain. Instead you just compact pain on top of pain.

Life at this point can get more and more complicated. Have you ever wondered why so many overweight, overeating people appear to be jolly? Many, never having been able to express feelings, become people pleasers who have little or no way to protect themselves emotionally from demands others place on them. But we need those shields that separate us from other individuals, and when all else fails, *excess weight can become that shield*.

But I Need to Eat!

It's all too easy to use food for anything *but* nourishment. There's a saying that some people "eat only to live," but how many of us secretly "live only to eat"? People who never touch alcohol, drugs or cigarettes often use food as their "vice," their real "pleasure" in life. Even people who have been able to give up smoking find food to be another story.

Actually, overeating becomes the way of life, with an addictive pull as strong as any other chemical substance. But we cannot abstain from food, as we can from other abused substances. Rather we must control it daily.

You see, food, like money, is not inherently evil. Humans *must* have it to survive! We were created to eat and to enjoy the tastes of food. We are *physically* dependent upon food to survive. The problems begin when we are *emotionally* dependent on food to cope with everyday life. Food becomes an evil when we love it and eating more than we love God, more than we love ourselves and more than we love others.

Food is evil when it becomes our "golden calf." As recorded in Exodus 32, God, Moses and the top of Mount Sinai seemed too remote and far away for the Israelites waiting in the valley below. Anxious for a quick-fix "god" that they could touch, that was close at hand, that could "go before them," they molded a calf of gold.

We likewise turn to food, because it's always there at hand, because it gives immediate gratification.

How often, when we face difficult circumstances, does God seem too far away? How often do we turn to another "god" (a chocolate bar, donuts, ice cream) to make us feel better? How often do we use food to "go before us" in an uncomfortable situation?

(Of course, like the golden calf, food is a false god. Our desire for an all-powerful God can be momentarily quenched with overeating, but never fulfilled. Eating can never satisfy or give us peace or take away the pain. It just adds more stress, because now we have guilt on top of the other emotions!)

It is the *love* of food, the *love* of eating, that snares us. We are trapped as prisoners when food becomes more to us than physical nourishment. It entraps us when we use food to meet emotional and spiritual needs.

I've been here myself. Even as a preteen I had a "Scarlett O'Hara" way of dealing with problems. ("I can't think about this today. I'll think about it tomorrow.") But I needed something to help me push that problem into tomorrow, and food fit the bill. By the time I was in college, food had become my emotional escape-hatch. I didn't have to wait on God if eating could make me feel better. I had become emotionally and spiritually dependent upon food. For me, relief was just a swallow away!

Food Dependent?

Yes, millions of Americans are emotionally dependent on food. What does that mean?

An eating dependence, or disorder, is an illness in that it is a destructive process with a set of characteristic symptoms that are beyond the control of an individual. Eating dependency has nothing to do with your present weight. You may be quite overweight or very thin. It is an illness in which food has assumed an unnatural importance in your life and has come to dominate the physical, emotional and spiritual you. It is an improper relationship with food that has life-damaging consequences.

Food is a trap when it is used as a substitute for love, friendship or success, or when it's used to cover up more serious emotional issues.

Amy no longer recognized the "thin girl" in her wedding pictures. She had started to gain weight soon after she married. She had quit her job as a kindergarten teacher to prepare for her marriage to Jim. After the romance and excitement of her wedding had settled down, she missed the encouragement and affirmation she'd received from the parents of her students and the sweet hugs only five-year-olds can give. And Jim—he no longer seemed to be as devoted to her as when they were dating. "I love you" rarely left his lips.

Amy turned to food to handle the loneliness and disappointments in her life. A vicious cycle began: The more she ate and the heavier she got, the more isolated she felt and the more she ate. The more she ate and the heavier she became, the more depressed she became, and she ate when she felt depressed.

The food trap ruins a person's health and causes untold guilt, suffering and anguish. This is not being overly dramatic: We are killing ourselves with food. We are cutting our days on this earth short, and we're robbing the life out of the days we are here.

As Jesus warned, "Be careful, or your hearts will be weighed down with dissipation, drunkenness and the anxieties of life, and that day will close on you unexpectedly like a trap" (Luke 21:34).

Many people, including Katie, whom I described at the beginning of the chapter, cover up their eating dependencies with pendulum swings in their weight. They can overcome overeating as long as they are walking in the iron-will discipline of a diet. To cope with emotions, they replace the obsessive use of food with obsessive dieting. The diet becomes their fuel. As long as they can mask their eating problems with periodic stabs at willpower, they can deny their real problems. If I just had more discipline or motivation, the problem—my weight—would go away!

But the struggle with food and weight only gets worse. With a fat-thin disorder, you will be intensely preoccupied with food most of the time. You will occasionally become excessively preoccupied with dieting and/or exercise routines and get your weight down. But ultimately you will have a lapse. For all your hard work you'll reward yourself with a donut. That momentary lapse puts you into the I've-blown-it-now syndrome, so you eat a dozen donuts.

You then tell yourself, "I've really blown it now, so hang the self-discipline. I'll diet tomorrow." "Eat today, diet tomorrow" becomes *"Eat a lot today—everything you can't have when you diet tomorrow."* It's almost a last-supper mentality. In short, a momentary *lapse* becomes a *relapse* and then another *relapse*, which ultimately leads to a *collapse*. You may justify your failure with excuses: "I'm just under too much stress right now"; "It's Christmas! Who could diet at Christmas?"; "Who wouldn't eat with a life like mine?"

An eating dependency is the result of a lifetime of complex issues. Each person is unique, and each person's situation is different. Some people have extremely painful and debilitating experiences with food and the emotions attached to it. Others don't and may be only mildly affected. Yet a common thread runs through all the experiences; it involves relationships with other people, ourselves and God.

A Look at Your Eating Patterns

For the next week keep a food diary, writing down everything you eat—and when you eat it. Also note any situations that make you uncomfortable, prompting you to turn to food even when not particularly hungry. A food diary should include the following: what you eat and when, thoughts, events and feelings.

This information will become invaluable as you read further and learn more about what a healthy relationship with food is all about.

TWO

BORN TO
BE FREE

Identifying the problem is the first step on the road to freedom. By naming the problem—whether it is using food to deal with emotions or being too dependent on food (or a compulsive eater or having an eating disorder or a food addiction)—you stop denying the problem. You meet it face to face. Like a lamp shining in the darkness, you illuminate the enemy. It is no longer an *unknown* enemy stalking you—with your not knowing when, where or how it will strike.

Until you name your illness, you will struggle with the belief that you are simply a "weak" person with no self-control or willpower. Many people suffering from eating illnesses spend their lives saying, "I *can* lose weight; I just have to make up my mind to do it!" "I know I can stick to this new diet; I'm getting started Monday morning." But again and again they can't. And for good reasons.

All of us desire change for our lives—genuine change. We try to commit to making that change, but we simply can't follow through on our commitment. We can make lists of what to do to try to change ourselves, but we remain powerless to break free from destructive patterns.

Experts in the field consider the twelve-step program of Alcoholics Anonymous (see appendix) to be the most successful for breaking free from any addictions and dependencies. Subsequent steps are built on Step One: coming to the realization that *you are powerless and that your life has become unmanageable.* Here in this foundational step, one starts to break denial and realize that he or she is entrapped and powerless to break free. One's dependency—whether it be on alcohol or food—is out of control or beyond the control of mere willpower.

Step Two is *coming to believe that a Power greater than yourself can restore you to sanity.* You have the power to choose to look to God for that power! You are trapped, strapped in an improper relationship with food, eating and your body; and the only way out is to find a new, proper relationship to fill the void. Food has been controlling you, and it's time to rise up and break its control with a power from on high.

Consider the power of God: If He could raise Jesus from the dead, He can surely help you break free from the food trap. Compulsive overeating is gluttony, and Jesus went to the cross so that you no longer need to be victimized by such compulsive behavior. He who lived above compulsions died so that you and I might be new creatures in Him, born again with spirits set free.

The Power Exchange

"In my anguish I cried to the Lord, and he answered by setting me free" (Ps. 118:5).

"The most powerful single force in the world is man's eternal desire to be free." While these insightful words of John F. Kennedy refer to political freedom, they ring true for every part of our lives. We have been designed and destined for a life-style of freedom. The Revolutionary War patriot Patrick Henry expressed this in a battle cry: "Give me liberty or give me death!"

Actually, a life without freedom *is* death—death to abundant living! Paul communicated this freedom cry when he wrote: "It is for freedom that Christ has set us free. Stand firm, then, and do not let yourselves be burdened again by a yoke of slavery" (Gal. 5:1).

No matter what popular thought may say, we are not born free; we are born to *be free*. Spiritual freedom comes with knowing God and His desires for our lives. "Say to the captives, 'Come out,' and to those in darkness, 'Be free!' " (Is. 49:9).

Anyone can have an intimate, personal relationship with the heavenly Father. He created us in His image and likeness. But we rebelled, and He designed a plan so that we need not be separated from Him. He who was perfect took on human form and came to earth, born of a woman. Jesus Christ, who never sinned, died an atoning death—He carried our sins to the grave—so that you and I could be forgiven of all sins. What's more, He arose from the grave—His power was stronger than death itself—so that you and I could have victory over negative and destructive forces. His power is ours when we accept His redeeming grace and ask His Spirit to live within us. God is not just a higher power that I am reaching up to. God in His love has reached down to us; He empowers us by living within us.

What do you need to do? Simply give your life to Him, making Him your Lord. When He is your Lord and Savior,

His Holy Spirit dwells within your spirit, linking your life with the unlimited power of God. It is the Holy Spirit who will guide and comfort you as you break free from the food trap.

One of the great paradoxes of the Christian faith is that no one is completely free until he or she has become totally submissive. "If you hold to my teaching, you are really my disciples. Then you will know the truth, and the truth will set you free" (John 8:31-32).

So often we try to get "cleaned up" before we come to God. We substitute a list of rules to change ourselves to get God to like us and accept us. God says, come as you are. "Come to me, all you who are weary and burdened, and I will give you rest" (Matt. 11:28). "Weary and burdened" means *as you are*. We say, "But You don't know what I've done." God says, come as you are. "But You don't know the *horrible* things I've done." God says, come as you are, "and I will give you rest." God has a gift to give you and me; we need only to turn around and receive it.

This simple prayer can change the course of your entire life: Father, thank You for creating me in Your image, in Your likeness. Thank You for providing a plan for adopting me into Your eternal family. In the name of Jesus I make Jesus the Lord of my life. I give my body, soul and spirit to You now. I receive Jesus as my Lord and Savior, and I choose to live my life by the power of the Holy Spirit. I choose to allow You to rule over every area of my life, including the area of eating and food dependency. I choose to love You and obey Your voice. In Jesus' name, amen.

Know that you now have a new powerhouse of strength within you. When you tap its resources you will soar with unreserved strength.

Do you not know?
  Have you not heard?
The Lord is the everlasting God,
  the Creator of the ends of the earth.
He will not grow tired or weary,
  and his understanding no one can fathom.
He gives strength to the weary
  and increases the power of the weak....
Those who hope in the Lord
  will renew their strength.
They will soar on wings like eagles (Is. 40:28-29,31).

I was awestruck when I learned that, in the original language, the word translated as *renew* means "exchange." Consider this: God does not just renew our human strength. He actually exchanges His power, His strength for ours! What a new perspective—to be operating with the strength of God.

But accepting Christ as Lord and Savior will not necessarily make the food trap spring open, releasing us as if by "magic." Note that our spirits are born anew, not our souls or emotions, which are the soil for unhealthy dependencies.

Renewal Is a Process

The people I see breaking free from the food trap acknowledge that they are three-part human beings—spiritual, emotional and physical. Breaking free encompasses all three areas. We can feel spiritually strong yet be emotionally wounded. We can feel emotionally wise but be in a spiritual vacuum. We can be "spiritually malnourished" from starving the spiritual person while feeding the physical body. We can be sick physically yet well spiritually. We can be held in the food trap for physical, emotional *or* spiritual reasons. Freedom means wholeness in body, soul and spirit.

Before I embraced nutrition as a profession, I was handicapped in all three areas of my life. I was searching for real answers to my questions about the purpose of life—my life. I knew I was spiritually empty, but I didn't have a clue as to how to "get filled." And with my "Scarlett O'Hara" way of dealing with emotions, I was carrying a lot of emotional baggage. Food had become the obvious way to fill up my spiritual vacuum; it was also fuel I needed to carry the emotional burden. So I was held captive spiritually, emotionally *and* physically.

As I learned more about nutrition and began to take care of my physical body, I became physically strong enough to overcome much of my abusive eating. But nutrition knowledge alone was not enough to free me from periodic binges and unhealthy eating. It was years later, when I gave control of my life to the Lord, before I could access the power to be truly free. It has required many more years to cease ignoring emotional wounds of my past and to receive healing!

Even if you've been a Christian for years, how many times have you found yourself doing the very thing that you hate? You and I have company! The apostle Paul admitted that he shared our common struggle in Romans 7:15: "I do not understand what I do. For what I want to do I do not do, but what I hate I do." He then goes on to identify the culprit: He was caught in the garments of his old man. Paul's spirit was born again; all things had become new But his soul—his mind—was still clothed with the old.

A few pages later the apostle Paul, writing to Roman Christians, said, "Do not conform any longer to the pattern of this world, but be transformed by the renewing of your mind" (Rom. 12:2). Our souls are transformed by the *renewing of our minds*, which is a process, not an overnight happening! As far as our emotions are concerned, we have to take off the old clothes and put on the new.

In Galatians 5:24 Paul said, "Those who belong to Christ Jesus have crucified the sinful nature with its passions and desires." You see, Jesus died for our sins. He died so that our passions and desires (the old mind) would be crucified. The things that used to control us have been crucified, but at any time we can take things off the cross and give them life again. The old man wants to live, wants to keep coming back

Once we receive the gift of God, the Holy Spirit, He begins the metamorphosis—the change in our lives—through the renewal of our minds. There is nothing automatic about the renewal of one's mind. We can stay stuck in the old patterns that we've developed to meet our emotional needs. If we've been using food to meet emotional needs, we can get stuck in that system. If we simply *love* food, we can continue to use it as a quick-fix. And if we feel guilty about our patterns, that guilt can serve as glue that keeps us "caught," because the guilt keeps us from admitting the underlying problems. Being caught in the food trap is being caught in our "old clothes"; we are trying to take them off, but our arms get stuck in the jacket.

Never think that you are powerless or "straitjacketed" so you cannot progress in your renewal. The mercy, compassion and power of the Lord Jesus Christ are your hope of restoration. He is the light that exposes darkness and brings forth the promise of the dawn. Paul made this cry: "What a wretched man I am! Who will rescue me from this body of death? Thanks be to God—through Jesus Christ our Lord!" (Rom. 7:24-25). With our freed spirits we are empowered by the God of creation to break free from our emotional trappings.

After making the decision to give your life to God, it's

important to continue to face yourself—your problems, sins, defects and dependencies. God wants to work in your life by bringing you into the truth—which makes you free. Living in the truth means facing the emotions, the pain, that we try to "stuff" with food. Remember, an eating disorder is an emotional dependency on food. Food has become more to us than physical nourishment.

We have grown accustomed to denying our pain and discomfort. During our early years, most of us found it necessary to shut down our feelings and "keep everything locked inside." We learned denial when expressing our own desires and needs caused rejection. As adults we find it difficult to accept the reality of our pasts, and these blind spots keep us from seeing the problems behind the unhealthy traps, such as overeating, that we have developed.

As we will see in later chapters, God wants to help you name the problem. He, the light of the world, serves as "a light shining in a dark place, until the day dawns and the morning star rises in your hearts" (2 Pet. 1:19). Open yourself to His light, His truth. As you read further, His Spirit in your spirit will bear witness to the truths you need to hear. However painful this may be, it is also the promise of the dawn!

PART II:

YOUR BODY: DESIGNED TO WORK FOR YOU, NOT AGAINST YOU

THREE

SETTING
THE STAGE

Most Christians know that spiritually they have been set free to live life abundantly. Some know that they have been set free to be fit and have freedom over food, and yet they don't see the fruit of that promise of freedom. They have prayed and been prayed for, but they have not been able to obtain their promised freedom.

I find that many of these people stumble because they are looking for a quick fix. They may be spiritually plugged in to God's power, but the light switch—of their physical and/or emotional systems—is turned off. In Part 2 of this book I want to introduce you to nutritional principles that, if used, will make your body work for you rather than against you.

Many of my patients find that as they become stronger physically—get their bodies on an even nutritional keel— they are free to move ahead and see the deeper level of emotional needs that hinder their health. Meeting the physical needs often gives the energy and motivation to deal with sometimes painful emotions that trigger their binging.

Learning How to Eat—Not Diet

Unlike the diet designers you may have followed in the past, I put more emphasis on *what* you should eat rather than what you have to avoid, on *when* you should eat and *why* you should be eating it. My goal is to help you learn how food plays a vital role in making the body work right.

These nutrition principles give the foundation for a "weigh" of life, with weight control and appetite control as a precious physical benefit. As your body begins to work *for you* rather than against you, it naturally helps you keep your appetite under control. If you feed the body in such a way as to keep it out of an extreme starvation mode, you allow it to burn fat, not muscle. If you keep your metabolism in a high gear, you burn calories and fats at an optimum rate. In doing this, certain foods benefit the physical you, and others, to be avoided, work as weapons against you.

Calories certainly *do* count in weight control, but how and when you eat those calories and where those calories come from are *most* important. By getting to know food in a new way, you've got a chance for establishing a friendship with it.

You *can* have control of your body, your energy level, your maximum healing ability and your own well-being! You can meet your physical body's natural need for food in an appropriate way, abstaining from compulsive eating or compulsive dieting. Thousands of people have done it, following the Ten Commandments of Good Nutrition presented in my books *Eat Well, Live Well* and *Alive and Well in the Fast Food Lane* (coauthored with Carolyn Coats).

Like the original "Big Ten," this set of simple principles,

here revised and updated, promises an abundant life. I designed these principles, which aim toward *physical* abundance, to cut through various controversies of nutrition and provide a frame on which to hang your changed perceptions about the place of food in your life.

Remember this: You don't need to learn how to diet; you need to learn how to eat.

The right perspective puts you on the path to healthful eating. You are not denying yourself. Instead you are choosing to give yourself a gift! Instead of focusing on foods to avoid, think about adding new, wonderful foods. You'll feel satisfied, not deprived, and you'll be so full of the best foods that you won't desire the ones that drag you down.

Making changes in eating behavior may seem as if it's taking on another duty or bondage. Actually, choosing to eat right foods at the right time is choosing freedom. Rather than binding you, self-control frees you to be the real you—free from binging, gluttony and overeating. You are in control of what goes into your body. You are healthier and more energetic.

The American Way

Over the years I've identified the typical pattern of eating in America (that comfortable land of the unhealthy). The pattern is a sorry reflection of our life-styles in terms of wellness. You see, America is winning lots of races, many that we've not bargained for. Globally we have the highest rates of obesity, heart disease and certain cancers. While we focus on our strength as a world power, our "people power" is being robbed of energy, vitality and life. Good health is part of our genetic heritage: God has scripted healing and repair into every molecule of DNA in the human body. The secret is to live so as to promote that healing and repair process rather than to hinder it.

Come with me as I look over the shoulder of a typical American on an average day.

Early A.M.: Most people report they have no time for breakfast or no interest in breakfast, or they just "aren't that hungry" in the morning. They start out with little or no breakfast—maybe a cup of coffee or diet soda on the run.

Some say that if they skip breakfast they don't get hungry until much later in the day. Eating seems to start some monster of an appetite, so it makes sense to push eating off as late as possible. Whatever the reason, most people don't eat much breakfast and do "just fine" until maybe ten o'clock.

10:00 A.M.: About now many feel a subtle dip in energy, a little twang that says, "Any donuts around? Any Danishes?" Someone is *always* celebrating something! Your scenario might go like this: If you can find something, you'll take it. But if nothing is available or you're too busy, you may be able to get by with another cup of coffee. If you're not a coffee drinker, you may have a diet soda to get that jolt of caffeine.

Lunch time: Like breakfast, lunch is not a priority meal for most Americans. Most do just fine with a burger on the run or cheese crackers from the vending machine or maybe something "healthy" like a salad. (Never mind the four hundred calories of blue cheese dressing; if it's a salad, it has to be good for you!)

Even if they feel a little drowsy right after lunch, almost drugged, they can push through and get a second wind. Actually, most Americans find they have pretty good energy and pretty good willpower and haven't been *that* hungry until the magic time of day called arsenic hour.

3:00 to 3:30 P.M. (arsenic hour): About now most people will eat anything and everything! This is the time when no matter how much energy they've had, no matter how unhungry they've been, it all falls apart. They whistle that little tune "Snickers is so satisfying," and the gorge begins.

However, if they're busy or food's not available, they may be able to push right through with another soda or cup of coffee—delaying arsenic hour until they get home.

Arrival home: Most of us walk in the door, do not pass go and head straight to the refrigerator. While we're deciding what, oh what, to have for dinner, or waiting for dinner to be served, we can eat an entire meal's worth of calories from the refrigerator. We have lots of "ration"alizations about eating at this time.

Food "Ration"alizations

- If I don't actually put food on a plate but eat straight from the containers in the refrigerator, the food doesn't count as calories. The "act" isn't premeditated, so I shouldn't be penalized for it.
- If I eat over the sink, those calories don't count either. Because I'm standing up, the food goes straight to my feet. It doesn't stop to be digested or absorbed, so it doesn't count against me.
- If I don't actually cut a brownie, but just "pick it to death," the calories won't count. I burn so many calories chewing so many small bites.
- If I taste the food while I'm cooking, those calories are "free." I'm just trying to assure the proper nutrition of my loved ones...such sacrificial work!
- If I eat the food left on the plates or serving dishes while I'm cleaning off the table, that won't count either. Those calories should count against that *wasteful person* who didn't clean the plate.

47

Dinnertime: When most people sit down for dinner, they may be half full, and by the time they have finished dinner, they *are* full—even stuffed. But as full as they may be, if they're the typical American, they are probably left with a vaguely dissatisfied feeling: If I just had something *sweet!* Just something....If there's nothing there, or if they're guilty enough about how much they've eaten, they may be able to ignore that sweet tooth.

8:30 P.M.: Many people have fallen asleep on the couch by this time. As a matter of fact, many don't know there is life after 8:30 at night; they sign off the air.

9:30 to 10:00 P.M.: If you've managed to stay awake past 8:30, you may settle down to watch some TV about now. A commercial comes on showing food so appealing you can almost smell and taste it. You hear a noise coming from the kitchen but ignore it because the show's coming back on. Then the next commercial comes, and the noise starts again. This time it's too loud to ignore; it's your responsibility to check it out. So you go peeking around the corner into the kitchen.

The freezer door is opening and closing, opening and closing, and a little round carton of ice cream is calling your name. It's the call of the wild. And the miracle is, a similar scene is happening all across the country.

Late every evening people hear a personal summons to the kitchen, and the typical day ends with that bowl of ice cream—or popcorn—or chips—or something!

The next day: You get up in the morning still full from the night before. You aren't really hungry for breakfast, aren't that interested in food in the morning, have no time to eat, until about ten o'clock—and the whole process repeats itself.

Good Intentions Gone Bad

This "day in the life" shows where most of us go wrong. The typical American eats little or nothing until that unmanageable time of day between 3:00 and 5:30 P.M., when no matter how strong we've been, how much energy we've had, how unhungry we've been, it all falls apart. During the "arsenic hour," control, self-discipline and willpower slip out of one's grasp. The calories start rolling in. Statistics indicate that most Americans eat 80 to 85 percent of a day's calories within a few concentrated hours.

Too Much, Too Late!

Regardless of the number of calories consumed, the body can use only a small amount of energy, protein and nutrients quickly. The rest is thrown off as waste or stored as fat. Eating in the typically American, lopsided way robs the body of vital nutrients for the remaining twenty hours, until the next evening. We not only go wrong in how much we eat or in what we eat; we also eat entirely *too much at the wrong time*.

The following Ten Commandments of Good Nutrition are not a magic formula to follow. They are just timeless truths that show you how the body was designed to work and how you can get food to work for you, not against you.

Do the best you can and aim for progress, not perfection!

FOUR

THE RIGHT THING AT THE RIGHT TIME

T he first three commandments focus on eating the right thing at the right time.

I

Thou Shalt Always
Eat a Protein With a Carbohydrate
(and Vice Versa)

The diets of our time have promised that eating either all proteins or all carbohydrates is *the* way to lose weight. But this kind of diet is designed to be out of balance. (There's a reason why they work so quickly and fail even more quickly!)

At every meal (and snack) eat a balance of carbohydrates and protein. The two kinds of food have two different

51

functions in your body. Carbohydrate is 100 percent pure energy. It's the fuel that burns. Protein, on the other hand, could be compared to bricks that build up a house's walls. Carbohydrates burn. Proteins build. That's if all goes well. If protein is eaten alone, the body will burn it as fuel, wasting it. (It is a less efficient source of energy.) The protein you eat needs to be protected so it can be used to build the new you.

Protein's building power. Protein is the new you! It makes muscles that shape your body; it makes new hair and new nails and beautifies your skin. It works to replace worn out cells and to regulate your body's functions and fluids. It boosts your metabolism. Protein is so important that you cannot be healthy (not even attractive) without it.

Protein is so powerful that we don't need very much of it; as a matter of fact, a six-and-one-half-ounce can of chicken provides all the protein you need for the whole day. "A little dab will do you" certainly applies to protein. The typical American diet provides us with two to three times the amount recommended.

The *amount* of protein you eat is not the main issue here. You see, protein is not stored, so it must be replenished frequently through the day, each and every day of your life. Never believe anybody who tells you that you don't need protein or that you should eat it only once a day. You are robbing your body of protein's healing and building power all day long.

But when off balance, things get even worse. Without carbohydrate, when protein and fat are used for energy, a waste product called ketones is thrown off.

This state of ketosis causes the body to dehydrate and lose a great deal of water weight. This is how a high-protein, low-carbohydrate diet can promise you a quick weight loss (such as ten pounds in ten days). Sadly, it's not fat that is lost; initially, it's water weight only. The scale does not have a measurement for fat, water or muscle weight; it gives simple poundage. We tend to play tricks with it. When we lose five pounds, we're just sure we've lost fat; if we gain five pounds, we're just sure we've gained water. The number on the scale can never be an accurate measure of progress. Water weight returns as quickly as it leaves.

What's what? The easiest way to think of "what's what" is to think of where it comes from. Anything that comes from a plant is carbohydrate, and anything that comes from an animal is complete protein. A miraculous exception to this is the *legume* family of plants (dried beans and peanuts) grown in the ground in such a way that they absorb nitrogen from the soil, becoming excellent sources of protein if eaten with a grain or a seed.

Unfortunately most of the popular protein foods are high in fat. And it's fat that makes us fat. It is also fat that sets us up for a myriad of killer diseases. By choosing the lower-fat versions of popular foods, we get all of protein's building power without the risks of fat.

Ideal Protein Sources

- nonfat milk and plain yogurt
- low-fat cheeses: farmer's, Laughing Cow reduced-calorie wedges; "light" cream cheese; 1 percent, low-fat cottage cheese; mozzarella; part-skimmed ricotta; any other part-skimmed milk cheese with less than five grams of fat per ounce
- eggs (particularly use the egg whites)
- fish and seafood
- chicken, turkey, cornish game hens, other poultry

- veal and lean, well-trimmed beef, pork and lamb
- legumes: black beans; garbanzo beans; great Northern beans; kidney beans; lentils; navy beans; peanuts and natural peanut butter; red beans; split peas; soybeans. (Although a plant food, legumes contain valuable protein if eaten with a grain—corn, wheat, rice, oats—or a seed—pumpkin, sunflower, sesame.)

Carbohydrates: Energy Starters

Complex Carbohydrate: the Grains

bread, cereals, crackers, pasta
rice and wild rice, oats
barley, grits

Complex Carbohydrate: the "Starchy" Vegetables

potatoes (white and sweet), peas, winter squash
turnips, black-eyed peas, lima beans
corn and parsnips

Simple Carbohydrate:
Fruits and Nonstarchy Vegetables

all fruits and any vegetable other than
the starchy vegetables listed above, such as
asparagus, broccoli, beets, Brussels sprouts, cabbage
cauliflower, celery, carrots, leafy greens, green
beans, mushrooms, onions, tomatoes
and zucchini

Remember, stay away from advice that tells you not to eat carbohydrate or protein or not to eat them together. You'll be robbing your body of carbohydrate's energy and protein's building power *all day long*.

II
Thou Shalt Never Skip Breakfast

Mom was right! Breakfast will make you feel better. Why? Because it helps you start your day with a metabolism in high gear and your appetite in control.

Think of the body as a campfire that dies down during the night. In the morning it needs to be stoked up with wood if it's to burn vigorously again.

The body awakens in a slowed, fasting state. The fuel is low, and what is there isn't being burned efficiently. As you "break the fast" with breakfast, you meet the body's demand for energy and boost the efficiency of the metabolic system.

What happens if you don't eat breakfast? The body turns to its own muscle mass (not fat!) for energy and slows down even more, conserving itself for the long haul of a "starved" state. Much later when you do eat, even "gorge," most of that food will have to be stored as fat because the body isn't burning energy fast enough to use the calories you've consumed. The fire has gone out. The food you eat is much like dumping an armload of firewood on a dead fire, and a lot of Americans are walking around with dead wood sitting on top of their fires.

No one saves calories by skipping breakfast. Eating breakfast gears up the metabolism, burning fuel (the calories) more efficiently. Thus, the calories you consume will be burned rather than stored.

I bet you've said this, "If I skip breakfast, I don't really get hungry till much later in the day. If I eat breakfast, I get hungry every few hours.''

You're right! If this is your pattern, your body is functioning properly. Here's how it works: When you starve in the morning, waste products are released into your system that temporarily depress your appetite and allow you to continue to starve without feeling hungry for hours.

But think it through. If this happens, *you're setting yourself up to overeat*; as soon as you begin to eat, your appetite is really "turned on." Because your blood sugar level has dropped so low, your physical body actually overrides your willpower to stop eating.

On the other hand, if you eat breakfast, your day begins right: You stabilize your blood sugars, which in turn gives you more energy, an increased ability to concentrate and an appetite that is under *your* control.

I always prided myself in not "having" to eat breakfast. No matter how out of control my eating may have been later in the day, breakfast was one meal I could control. I could always start each day being "above food." Besides, I knew I was going to overeat later in the day, so it made sense to cut calories where I could! I was teaching nutrition at a college level before I came face-to-face with the reality of the importance of breakfast. I tried and tried to get by without it, but each time I skipped, I saw that I was operating that day with an energy handicap. I never had the supply to meet the demands! The demands continued, of course, and I met them; but I was paying the price with my moods, my clarity of thinking and my energy. Inevitably I would overeat in the afternoon or evening to make up for what had been depleted.

Most people skip breakfast because they "don't have time" to fix it and eat it. But no one is saying that breakfast has to be a time robber. You can fix it quickly and eat it "on the run" if you must.

Remember, breakfast is the "stick" that stokes the metabolic fire.

Of course a breakfast needs to supply adequate carbohydrate and protein. Breakfast should never be just a piece of toast. It should be toast *with* cheese—or an egg—or natural peanut butter—or yogurt. It might be cereal with milk, another breakfast choice that provides the body with carbohydrates to burn and proteins to build.

III

Thou Shalt
Eat a Healthy Meal or Healthy Snack
Every Three to Four Hours and
Have Your Healthy Snack Handy

Once you've started the day with breakfast, stabilizing your body first thing in the morning, your eating goal is to keep your blood sugars up and even.

Blood sugar normally crests and falls every three to four hours. As it falls, your energy will fall right with it—along with your mood, your concentration and your ability to handle stress. But one thing soars—your physical appetite for food. As your blood sugar drops, every cell in your body sends a signal to your brain demanding to be fed. And the signal is not requesting broccoli; it's screaming for a quicker source of energy. The brain equates that with chocolate, chips or whatever food happens to be your "special friend." If, at the same time, emotional messages are playing through your mind, signaling an eating response, you are apt to fall head first into overeating.

By never letting your blood sugar "fall," rather undergirding it with small amounts of food evenly spread through the day, you will be able to keep your *physical* appetite in control. Because you are eating right things at the right time, you're not as apt to fall into wrong things at the wrong time. Because you're meeting your needs physically, your desires can change. Balanced eating calls for many changes in the "all-American" diet. We've grown up with a three-square-meals mentality, with the idea that snacking is nutritional enemy number one. Snacks *are* the enemy, if you're thinking of potato chips, ice cream, candy bars and sodas. This type of snacking can be nutritionally and calorically disastrous, providing high amounts of fat, sugars and salt and little or no nutritional value.

But you *can* enjoy healthy snacks; you can actually *put snacking to use for you.* Use it to prevent your blood sugar from dropping too low, leaving you sleepy and craving sweets. Think in terms of power snacking, using snacks to arm you with control.

Keep a log on the fire. Not only will several small meals throughout the day keep your appetite in control; it will keep your body in a higher rate of metabolism. Remember the campfire story? Healthy snacking is very much like throwing wood on a fire all through the day. Your body was created to survive, and it reads those long hours without food as starvation. It will dramatically slow down rather than burn your valuable muscle mass. Contrary to what many think, in a starvation state when no carbohydrate is available, your body turns first to muscle mass for energy and last to your fat stores. To metabolize calories efficiently, burning them for energy rather than burning muscle, feed your body the right thing at the right time.

Smaller, more frequent meals will provide more energy, more healthy weight loss and easier weight maintenance. Several small meals a day deposit less fat than one or two large meals, even if you eat the same food and in the same amount.

Plan your meals to include three meals and at least one snack per day. By planning your eating to include a certain number of meals at certain times of the day, you gain freedom from almost continuous obsession about whether you should eat now and, if so, what and how much. Generally, I plan to eat 25 percent of the day's calories at breakfast, 25 percent at lunch, 25 percent at dinner and the remaining 25 percent as healthy snacks throughout the day.

Always have those healthy snacks handy. When you don't have good choices available, you're likely to reach for an unhealthy snack or not eat at all for an extended time. Either scenario will set you up for disaster later on in the day. Do what I do: Keep healthy snacks in your car, in your desk drawer, in your briefcase—wherever you may find yourself at those critical "down" times. This is not food dependency; it actually frees you from out-of-control eating. It is using food wisely to meet the body's physical need—the supply to meet the demand.

Some Examples of Power Snacks

- whole grain crackers and low-fat cheese
- rice cakes and natural peanut butter
- fresh fruit and cheese
- plain yogurt blended with fruit or one of the new all-fruit jams
- whole grain cereal with skimmed milk
- popcorn sprinkled with Parmesan cheese
- oat bran muffin with skimmed milk
- small pop-top can of water-packed tuna with whole grain crackers

- a "trail mix" of unsalted peanuts, unsalted shelled sunflower seeds and raisins. (This trail mix is a favorite snack and an easy one. Make it in abundance and bag up into one-quarter-cup batches. *In this amount*, this balanced snack provides the good fiber and protein of peanuts but not too much of their fat and calories.)

Take control of your appetite. Food through the day keeps a ravenous appetite away! Your blood sugar level is the system for controlling your physical appetite. I have most of my patients keep their blood sugar even by eating every two-and-a-half to three hours. This enables their bodies never to get too hungry, so they are satisfied much more quickly, with much less food.

Though schedules do not always allow us to eat leisurely, for several reasons I recommend that eating meals or snacks be a separate dining experience that takes place while sitting at a table, not standing over the sink. Eating over the sink or in front of an open refrigerator does not equate with dining satisfaction—only mindless on-the-run eating. (And eating in front of the television can make TV watching become an emotional trigger for eating.)

We Americans tend to eat too fast, and this contributes to our lack of appetite control. Our appetite for food is satisfied by a "triggering" system in which the body tells the brain, "I am full. Stop eating!" But this is a delayed trigger that takes twenty to twenty-five minutes to kick in. By continuing to eat in a fast and frenzied style, we can consume enormous quantities of food before we ever feel satisfied. *Slow down your eating and give your body a chance for* natural *portion control.*

Dining, Rather Than Eating

Here are four tips that will help control your appetite as you dine at meals:

- Eat fruit as an appetizer rather than as dessert. This simple carbohydrate will start raising your blood sugar, allowing your appetite regulator to be satisfied by the time you are finishing your meal. Fruit as appetizer will also prevent the drowsiness that often follows a meal; its natural sugar is released as energy into the blood stream quickly (within fifteen or twenty minutes).

- Serve salad or raw vegetables as your second course. This will "slow down" the meal itself and provide bulk that will dull your appetite.

- Completely chew and swallow before putting more food on the fork. We are often so busy shoveling the food in that we don't realize we have our forks, poised and ready, at our mouths while we're still chewing the prior bite. Practice putting your fork down at least every third bite.

- Eat your smaller protein portion intermittently between the other items on your plate. Subconsciously we tend to feel that once our meat is gone, we are only "finishing up."

Remember, to prevent the "sinking syndrome" in the late afternoon and evening, eat a balance of carbohydrate and protein evenly through the day. If your physiological needs are met by feeding your body properly, *your desires for food change*; where there is less need, you have more control over desire.

Iron-will discipline has never controlled food intake and never will. No checklist or rigid diet plan will enable that control. If our blood sugar level drops, our cells will send messages to our brains saying, "Feed me!" Time and again the body will override willpower. "He who is full loathes honey, but to the hungry even what is bitter tastes sweet" (Prov. 27:7). Remember whose power is helping you take control; He can succeed where all others have failed.

FIVE

MORE OF
THE BEST, LESS
OF THE REST

The next four commandments focus on the foods and nutrients that benefit the body, allowing it to work for you in an optimal way. The goal here is to *have more of the best and less of the rest!*

IV
Thou Shalt
Double Your Fiber

Grandma used to say, "Eat your roughage." Now, years later, the surgeon general has said, "Double your fiber." This can be done rather easily, not with fiber pills but with wholesome foods prepared in a wholesome way. Whole grain breads and cereals, unprocessed oat and wheat bran, legumes, fresh fruits and fresh vegetables are wonderful foods loaded with wonderful fiber.

Fiber is the part of plants not digested by the body. There are two types of fiber. The *water soluble* fibers—found in the gum and pectin of fruits, oats, barley, brown rice and legumes—lower cholesterol levels and help control blood sugar levels. The *water insoluble* fibers—found in all whole grains, fresh vegetables and wheat bran—are an excellent means of controlling bowel problems such as constipation, diarrhea and diverticulosis.

To keep the body working at its best, we need both soluble and insoluble fibers. The soluble fiber adds bulk and softness to the stool, and the insoluble moves it along. But fiber needs lots of wonderful water to activate it, ideally eight to ten glasses a day.

Research links an insufficient intake of fiber to the prevalence of our killer diseases: heart disease, obesity, cancer and diabetes. The continuing rise in these diseases may be, in part, connected to the food industry's *refining* of their products.

Refinement and enrichment: a robbery that's legal. Consider this story: A man is walking down the street when he is approached by a robber.

The thief forces the man at gunpoint to take off everything he is wearing—everything! After the man strips, the thief says, "I have just refined you."

He then proceeds to return only four things—the man's watch, one shoe, his undershirt and necktie—and proclaims, "I have just enriched you."

Returning four nutrients and leaving out twenty-one is what this enrichment thing is all about. When a whole wheat berry is refined, every nutrient is affected (twenty-one are completely lost), and all of its protective fiber is stripped away. In the enrichment process, only four nutrients are added back. Don't be fooled by advertisements! White, refined carbohydrate, even though it's enriched, is never nutritionally as good as whole grain.

Compared to refined grains, whole grains will better satisfy and control your appetite and energy level. Why? Because the fiber acts something like a time-release capsule, slowly and evenly releasing food sugars into your system. By preventing a rapid rise and dramatic fall of the blood sugar level, by providing more bulk and by staying in the stomach longer, whole grain foods will work for you as you try to gain control over your appetite.

How Do I Double My Fiber?

- Use whole grains, such as brown rice, oats and *whole* wheat rather than the white, refined types. When purchasing, look for labels that indicate 100 percent whole wheat with the word *whole* being first in the ingredient list.

  Many manufacturers call products "whole grain" even if they contain only minimal amounts of bran. Brown dye does wonders at making foods *look* healthy!
- Eat vegetables and fruits with well-washed skins.
- Choose more raw or lightly cooked vegetables in as nonprocessed a form as possible.

  As food becomes processed, ground, mashed, pureed or juiced, the fiber effectiveness is decreased.
- Add a variety of legumes to your diet.

V

Thou Shalt
Believe Your Mother Was Right:
Eat Your Fruits and Veggies

Vegetables and fruits provide a storehouse of vitamins, minerals, flavors and pigments that serve as protectors against disease. They are also valuable sources of fiber and fluid. They are satisfying munchies that make up an enormously healthy part of a healthy diet.

Vegetables and fruits: great cancer fighters. Research shows that the very substance that makes broccoli, broccoli— or cauliflower, cauliflower—has cancer preventative properties. This flavoring substance is found only in vegetables belonging to the cruciferous family (cabbage, cauliflower, broccoli and Brussels sprouts). Try to eat one of these cooked or raw every day. You'll even get an extra bonus in their vitamin C content, as studies are showing this blocks the action of certain body chemicals that lead to cancer and heart disease.

Beta-carotene, one of the substances responsible for the vivid coloring in fruits and vegetables, appears to block the process by which a normal cell turns malignant. Beta-carotene is found in fruits and vegetables with a deep yellow-orange or dark green color. The body converts this pigment to vitamin A, though never in toxic amounts. Eating these wonderful vegetables and fruits is the safe, miraculous way for us to obtain vitamin A.

Color magic. You may not be able to tell a book by its cover, but you can surely choose a fruit or vegetable by its color. Generally, the more vivid the color, the higher it is in essential nutrients. That deep orange-red coloring in carrots, sweet potatoes, cantaloupes, apricots and strawberries means vitamin A. Dark green, leafy vegetables, such as greens, spinach, romaine lettuce, Brussels sprouts and broccoli, are also loaded with vitamin A, as well as folic acid.

Vitamin C is found in more than just citrus. It is power-packed into strawberries, cantaloupe, tomatoes, green peppers and broccoli. Remember, if they're loaded with color, they're loaded with nutrition.

Cookin' good!. Bringing nutritious foods home from the market is just the start. The way you cook them matters, too. Cooking affects not only the taste and appearance of the food, but also the nutritional value.

Tips to Retain Vegetables' Valuable Vitamins

- Buy vegetables as fresh as possible. When fresh is not possible, frozen is the best alternative. (Avoid those frozen with butter or sauces.)
- Use well-washed peelings and outer leaves of vegetables whenever possible. That's where the highest concentration of nutrients is found. Wash vegetables in water with a few drops of dish-washing detergent added. Don't peel your vegetables, unless the food is waxed; it's a waste of time and nutrients.
- Store vegetables in airtight containers in the refrigerator.
- Do not store vegetables in water. Too many vitamins are lost.
- The best cooking techniques are steaming, microwave cooking, stir-frying or pressure cooking. Cook only till crisp-tender.

VI

Thou Shalt
Get Your Vitamins and Minerals
From Food, Not Pills

Vitamins are organic molecules that the body cannot produce on its own but yet cannot do without. As chemical catalysts for the body, they make things happen. Vitamins do not give energy, but they help the body convert carbohydrates to energy and then they help the body use that energy.

Minerals, unlike vitamins, are inorganic compounds. Some minerals become building blocks for structures such as bones and teeth. Others work with the fluids of the body, giving them certain characteristics. We consume only small amounts of minerals daily, compared to the amount of vitamins in our diet. Some thirty minerals are important in nutrition.

Any varied diet with enough calories should provide the essential vitamins and minerals the body needs. The majority of people do not need to take artificial vitamins in a pill form or as part of "fortified" products. Rather than using blanket supplementation, try to improve your eating patterns to assure adequate intake of all nutrients. The best source of vitamins and minerals is, and always has been, *food!*

Vitamins are either fat-soluble or water-soluble. Fat solubles (A, D, E and K) are absorbed through the intestinal walls and can be stored in the body fat for long periods of time. Because they accumulate in the body, you can get into a toxic state from taking megadoses or amounts that are more than ten times the RDA (recommended daily allowance). In this mega-amount the vitamins are no longer being used as vitamins but as drugs, carrying side effects of drugs. Most people are not aware of this when they start taking megadoses of vitamins. They figure that, if a little is good, a lot is better.

Some minerals are stored like the fat-soluble vitamins and, like them, are toxic if taken in excess. These are iron, copper, choline, magnesium, manganese, iodine and fluorine. Other minerals do not appear to accumulate in the body and are readily excreted, so toxicity is not as great a risk.

At best, using vitamins or minerals as a sort of insurance policy is a waste of money. At worst, they can be highly toxic.

Water-soluble vitamins (B complex and C) cannot be stored in the body for long because they dissolve in water and are released in the urine. Although at one time these were considered harmless in megadoses, some studies now show that large quantities of even these water-soluble vitamins, over a period of time, can lead to problems. B-6 and niacin are two such vitamins that have been marked as dangerous in megadoses.

When it comes to minerals, three are major problems in the American diet. We get far too much sodium and far too little calcium and iron. Iron and calcium merit special attention—iron because 20 percent or more of American women have severely low iron stores and may be suffering from iron deficiency anemia, and calcium because of women's high risk of osteoporosis. (See page 85 for ways to pass up the salt!)

Who needs vitamins and minerals? *Every human being.* Who would need a vitamin and mineral supplement? Those at high risk of a vitamin-mineral deficiency: chronic dieters whose nutrition gets cut with their calories; the chronically ill; heavy drinkers and smokers; pregnant women and nursing mothers; those who have a limited choice of food intake. In these cases, a basic multivitamin and mineral supplement that supplies no more than 150 percent of the RDA (recommended daily allowance) would be advised.

No single food supplies your daily requirement of all the vitamins and minerals. There is no one perfect food. Many trace vitamins and minerals are found in small quantities in a few foods. Actually foods may contain nutrients that we still know nothing about. Eating a variety of foods in their whole form provides you with the whole gamut of vitamins and minerals, possibly including as yet hidden benefits.

The beautiful thing about good, balanced nutrition is this: Everything fits together in such a perfect way that just focusing on these ten basic principles will allow adequate intake of essential nutrients. You don't have to be continually analyzing your intake to be sure you've had your zinc today.

Breaking the rut. I've discovered that some of the benefits of a varied diet are emotional. For many people, eating healthily means eating in a rut—a boring rut. We settle into a limited variety of dishes in which we feel "safe" and don't have to make any choices. We don't want to give much thought to what we're going to eat. It's just easier to have a bowl of the same cereal for breakfast, a "ditto" turkey sandwich for lunch and piece of chicken for dinner.

Why such a rut? It's easier to trust the rut than to trust ourselves to make healthy choices. Then we may subconsciously be trying to work "magic," thinking that just the right (the only) combination of food will work for us. Some people seem to punish themselves with the same old boring foods, thinking they are paying some penance for their last binge. Some, not caring enough about themselves to do anything differently, feed themselves with as much forethought and effort as their dogs.

Time and again I've seen that ruts cause problems, setting patients up to overindulge as soon as they get the taste of anything more exciting. Then once they get off track, it becomes very difficult to get back on track—since "on track" means returning to the same old boring rut!

Healthy eating doesn't need to be anything less than enjoyable, tasty and full of variety.

Chapter 12 of this book includes complete meal plans and recipes. Try them—to get free from your eating rut.

Anemic? Not me! Studies have shown that the overwhelming majority of women take in less iron than their bodies require. Again, more than 20 percent of American women are at high risk of anemia, particularly during their menstrual flows. Men are generally not in such danger, except when they may have blood loss from a disease (such as ulcers) or from dieting in such a way that robs their bodies of valuable iron and protein. To prevent this anemia, women should take in as much iron as possible through dietary sources.

Eating evenly through the day, never overloading the body at any one time with iron, allows the body to absorb iron more effectively. Iron is a mineral that the more you put in at one time, the less the body absorbs. That's why eating smaller amounts of food more frequently helps to fight anemia. Also, when an iron supplement is called for, splitting up the amount into two doses is valuable.

It is not uncommon for women who eat a well-balanced diet to require additional iron, especially when their caloric intake is restricted for weight loss. Your needs can be confirmed by getting a hemoglobin or hematocrit check, which shows the iron stores in your cells. If you are anemic or on the borderline, try a well-absorbed iron supplement for at least six to eight weeks and make positive changes in your eating patterns. If additional iron is called for, the best over-the-counter form is *ferrous gluconate*. One brand name of this is Fergon.

Food Sources High in Iron

- lean meats and poultry
- oysters and clams
- whole grains and cereals
- dried fruits
- legumes (dried beans and peanuts)
- dark green, leafy vegetables

Eating Tips to Fight Anemia

- Eat small, frequent meals throughout the day.
- Always eat a carbohydrate with a protein, as protein enhances your iron absorption.
- Eat fruits high in vitamin C (citrus, strawberries and pineapple) and vegetables from the cabbage family (broccoli, cabbage and cauliflower) at your meals and snacks, as vitamin C enhances your absorption of iron.
- Avoid drinking tea, colas and coffee with your meals or snacks, as these contain tannic acid which *hinders* your absorption of iron. Drink wonderful pure water instead.

Ammunition to fight osteoporosis. Osteoporosis is a painful and crippling loss of bone mass that usually begins earlier in life but worsens after menopause. It is eight times more common in women than in men and is characterized by stooped posture, loss of height and an increased risk of fractures. Although this disease is seen commonly in the elderly, *it is not a normal part of aging*. It can be prevented. The ammunition: calcium and exercise, along with proper hormonal balance.

Women have a particularly high need for calcium for three reasons: They mature faster and earlier than men, resulting in a lower bone density; pregnancy, nursing and menopause increase the need for calcium; many women miss out on proper exercise, which helps build stronger bones.

Recent studies show that most women don't get half the calcium they need. Unfortunately, osteoporosis can be the pay-later penalty for skimping on calcium now.

The condition starts in the midthirties with symptoms first appearing in the midfifties and early sixties. The hormonal change at menopause speeds up the bone loss. Adequate calcium in the earlier years can help you build stronger bones to diminish your chances of osteoporosis later on. Adequate calcium in your later years can help halt the process.

All people need calcium throughout their lives, about eight hundred milligrams or three servings of a high-calcium food each day. Growing children and pregnant women have higher needs, requiring twelve hundred milligrams of four servings of high-calcium food a day. Women over thirty-five, however, need fourteen hundred milligrams of calcium, or five servings. This is a difficult requirement to meet from dietary sources alone, and calcium supplements may be necessary.

What Foods Are High in Calcium?

One serving

Dairy products*

Milk or plain yogurt . . . . 1 cup
Cheese . . . . 1-1/2 ounces
Cottage cheese . . . . 1-1/2 cups
Part-skim ricotta cheese . . . . 1/2 cup

Salmon, canned . . . . .5 ounces
Collard or turnip greens . . . . 1 cup
Broccoli . . . . .2 cups
Tofu or fortified soy milk . . . . 1 cup
Dried beans, cooked . . . . 2-1/2 cups

*The calcium content will be the same in whole, low-fat or
skimmed milk products, but low-fat products are suggested for
overall health.

Calcium supplements are sometimes recommended as
additions to a balanced diet for those people with especially
high needs. If you require supplements, consider these four
facts: (1) Calcium carbonate and calcium citrate are the best
absorbed forms. (2) Calcium will be better absorbed when
taken with a meal or small snack. (3) Your body makes the
best use of calcium taken at bedtime. (4) Two calcium
preparations, dolomite and bone meal, have occasionally been
found to be contaminated with lead and *should be avoided*.

VII

Thou Shalt
Drink at Least Eight
Glasses of Water a Day

Water makes up 92 percent of your blood plasma, 80 percent of your muscle mass, 60 percent of your red blood cells
and 50 percent of everything else in your body. What an
important ingredient to good health. Water, often ignored,
is as essential a nutrient as the other five: carbohydrates, proteins, fats, vitamins and minerals.

Being *the* natural diuretic, it prevents excess fluid retention.
Water helps to maintain proper muscle tone, allowing

muscles to contract. It also works to keep the skin healthy and resilient.

Being a mild laxative, water allows proper bowel function and waste elimination. It actually activates the fiber you eat to aid in digestion. Water is the vehicle the body must have to flush out the waste produced in normal body functions. Many other beverages, although water-based, contain substances the body has to work to metabolize or excrete. Caffeine in coffee is a diuretic, actually removing more water than is in the coffee itself. Beyond the caffeine in tea, the tannic acid is a waste product that competes for excretion with the waste products the body produces. The colorings and chemicals in diet sodas require the body to work to process and excrete them. Even juices do not provide the benefits of pure, wonderful water. Although you may drink other beverages, do not let them become a poor substitute for the beverage your body likes best.

You need eight to ten glasses of water each day. As you begin to meet this need by drinking more water, your natural thirst for it will increase. Water drinking is habit forming; the more you drink, the more you want!

Try filling a two-quart container with water each morning and make sure it's all gone before going to bed. If you are drinking tap water, the taste will likely improve with refrigeration for twenty-four hours. (The chlorine dissipates.) Purified or bottled water is a nice treat and is particularly refreshing with lemon or lime slices. Drinking water through a straw adds enjoyment for many.

We probably all know someone who gives water the credit for their good health. Because so many of us struggle with bodies that are working sluggishly, increasing our water intake to meet the body's needs *can* seem to produce some quite miraculous results. As Americans, most of us grew up drinking just about anything *but* water—soda, tea, coffee, punch, Kool-Aid—and water was only what we took pills or brushed teeth with. When we drink water properly along with eating nutritious foods, the body simply works as it was created to work.

SIX

DENTS IN
YOUR ARMOR

The previous commandments for good nutrition have focused on the patterns and nutrients vital to wellness. The last three commandments address foods and substances to be avoided. These do not benefit the body and can even cause serious health problems if taken to excess. They serve as weapons against your body and well-being, and, in the case of sugar and caffeine, they can easily lead you to over-indulgence.

When we eat for wellness, it's easy to see how our bodies were created. The body so reinforces the positive changes that the past negative eating patterns lose much of their value. Why eat foods that rob us of health, energy and well-being? When you feel good, really good, physically, you want to hold onto the good health.

If you are taking in any or all of these substances to excess, if you have a "the more I have, the more I want" syndrome, these commandments are for you.

VIII
Thou Shalt
Trim the Fat From Your Diet

In Leviticus 3:17 a loving God gives a rather strong command for the well-being of His people: "This is a lasting ordinance for generations to come, wherever you live: You must not eat any fat...." It should be no surprise when, thousands of years later, "modern science" discovers the link between disease and the consumption of fat. Consider these facts:

- Excess fat intake increases your cholesterol and your risk of heart disease and stroke.
- Excess fat intake increases your risk of cancer, particularly of the colon and breast.
- Excess fat intake increases your risk of gall bladder disease.
- Excess fat, particularly saturated fat (animal fat and coconut and palm oil), has been shown to elevate blood pressure, regardless of the person's weight.
- Excess fat fed to animals with a genetic susceptibility to diabetes made them far more likely to develop the disease. (People with a family history of diabetes could cut their fat consumption as a preventative measure against this disease.)
- Excess fat makes you fat!

As much as we need to eat carbohydrates and proteins at each meal, we *don't* need fat in the quantities we consume. Yes, carbohydrates burn and proteins build, but it's *fat that makes you fat!*

One ounce of fat supplies twice the number of calories as one ounce of carbohydrate and protein, and research shows that fats in food are stored as fat on the body much more readily than these other two nutrients. It's not the bread and potatoes that provide damaging calories; it's the butter and mayonnaise we plop on top.

On the average, Americans derive too many of their calories from fat—some 40 to 45 percent rather than the recommended 25 to 30 percent. (One gram of fat has nine calories, one teaspoon of fat—five grams—forty calories.) A typical adult eats the fat equivalent of a stick of butter a day! Not me, you may say, yet chances are you are eating a lot more than you realize. Less fat in your diet means less fat on your body and less cholesterol in your blood.

Most women should take in approximately forty grams of fat per day (or less). This means eight teaspoons. Most men should take in fifty grams of fat per day (or less, which means ten teaspoons).

In fighting fat your first line of defense is identifying your enemies. The main sources of dietary fat are meat, poultry, dairy products, nut foods and butter and oil toppings. Choosing the low-fat proteins on page 53 and preparing them in the low-fat methods will be small steps that make a big fat difference. Beautiful fruits, vegetables and grains have little fat as long as they are not fattened up with butters and sauces.

Small Steps That Make a Big Fat Difference

- Use skimmed milk, nonfat yogurt, skimmed milk cheese, low-fat cottage cheese and "light" cream cheese in place of any higher-fat dairy product.

- Eat more fish and white meats and fewer red meats. If you use red meats, buy lean and trim well—before *and* again after cooking. Cook them in a way that diminishes fat.
- Remove skin from poultry *before* cooking; you will cut the fat by 50 percent!
- Nonstick sprays and skillets enable you to brown meats without grease. Saute ingredients in stocks and broths rather than fats and oils to reduce the fat content of your recipes.
- If a recipe calls for basting with butter, adapt by basting with tomato or lemon juice or stock.
- Use canola or olive oil for salads or cooking. Small amounts of these oils are the most heart-healthy. You can also cut the oil called for in a recipe by two-thirds. For example, a recipe calling for three tablespoons of oil may be cut to one tablespoon. Ideally no more than one teaspoon of oil per serving should be used.
- Recipes calling for sour cream or mayonnaise will usually work if you substitute nonfat yogurt or blended-till-smooth low-fat cottage cheese or part-skimmed ricotta. These make a great topping for baked potatoes, especially sprinkled with chives or grated Parmesan.
- Purchase tuna packed in water rather than oil.
- Try using legumes (dried beans and peas) as a main dish or a meat substitute for a high-nutrition, low-fat meal.
- Use two egg whites in place of one whole egg. Egg whites are pure protein, and egg yolks are pure fat.
- Refrigerate soup stocks, meat drippings and

sauces, and remove the hardened surface layer of fat before reheating.

- If you use margarine, the soft, squeeze-type made of corn oil is best. Less preferable is tub margarine. Least preferable is stick. The firmer the margarine, the more saturated and unhealthy it is.

- Rarely, if ever, eat organ meats, such as liver, sweetbreads and brains. They are loaded with cholesterol.

- Use only *natural* peanut butter. Avoid commercial peanut butter at all costs, as it is not much more than shortening and sugar. Fresh-ground natural peanut butter still contains fat, but it is a great source of healthy protein. If you have trouble switching from the commercial type, begin by mixing it half and half with natural. Gradually increase the proportion of the natural until you have abandoned the commercial altogether.

- Remember that one of the most deceptive places for fat is in meals eaten away from home. The typical restaurant meal will contain the equivalent of twelve to fourteen pats of butter from the fats in the sauces, dressings, toppings and spreads. Get fats "to the side," and choose to apply them in small quantities.

IX

Thou Shalt
Consume a Minimum of
Sugar, Salt and Caffeine

Paul told the Corinthians, " 'Everything is permissible for

me'—but not everything is beneficial. 'Everything is permissible for me'—but I will not be mastered by anything" (1 Cor. 6:12).

In the American diet, sugar, salt and caffeine have become the big three—the cords that bind us in slavery. But, like Paul, we needn't be mastered by them. Let's look at the culprits one at a time.

Sugar: how sweet it isn't! Wise Solomon knew something about sweets: Proverbs 25:16 says, "If you find honey, eat just enough—toomuch of it, and you will vomit." Called by any name—honey, brown sugar, corn syrup, molasses, fructose—sugar is sugar!

Our problem with sugar is exacerbated because hidden sugars are found in nearly every packaged product on the grocer's shelf. If you have been raised on a typical American diet, you have been raised on a diet high in simple sugars and refined carbohydrates. Consider that the average can of soda contains eleven to twelve teaspoons of sugar, and you can see the overwhelming quantities of sugar the typical American consumes. One hundred and thirty-two pounds per year!

"But," you say, "I just have a sweet tooth." Actually, we all have a sweet tooth; we've been created with a natural preference for foods that taste sweet. Problems arise when this "natural" preference takes on an "unnatural" drive, fueled by a lifetime of poorly chosen foods and erratic eating patterns.

The health problems associated with sugar are controversial. On one side, voices call it "white death"; others cite few problems and see it as empty calories.

But sugar abuse *is* a threat to your well-being. It has been shown to cause dental cavities, obesity and high triglycerides, and it wreaks havoc in the control of diabetes and hypoglycemia. Unfortunately, healthy foods (such as fruit) that would contribute vitamins, minerals and fiber are often replaced by sugary foods, to the point at which deficiencies arise. Nutrient deficiencies spell malnutrition. In addition, most high-sugar snacks (candy bars, cookies, donuts, and the like) are loaded with saturated fats and calories.

Even occasional consumption of high-sugar foods is impossible for some, and it's not healthy for anyone. Those sensitive to blood sugar fluctuations can be hurt by "just a little bit"; sugar's seesaw effect seems to result in a "the more I have, the more I want" syndrome, laying the foundation for sugar abuse.

Here's how it works: A heavy sugar intake causes a pleasurable quick rise in blood sugar that is followed by a quick fall a few hours later. This dip in blood sugar triggers you to eat "for a lift" to relieve fatigue. You usually turn to something high in sugar again, and the up-and-down "seesaw" continues. If sweets aren't available, the affected blood sugar will make you feel vaguely dissatisfied with anything else. "If I just had something sweet..." seems to linger in your mind. Couple this sensation with erratic eating patterns, and eating can get out of hand. In some people even a small amount of concentrated sugar foods can cause strong enough blood sugar fluctuations to set the craving process in motion.

As mentioned earlier, continuous choosing of refined, highly concentrated sugar foods prevents us from choosing other nutrient-rich foods. The resulting nutrient-poor (junk) diet is often most to blame for the ill effects we see from a high-sugar diet. Many nutrients are easily lost in a "junk" diet: Iron, chromium and thiamine are just a few. The absence of these nutrients will result in a wide range of effects on personality, attention span, intellectual performance, sleep patterns, gastrointestinal function, and energy levels. Our tendency is to blame the "junk food," but it's most likely the "junk diet" (the lack of *good* food) that is to blame.

You may find it necessary to "withdraw" from the use of sweets to allow your blood sugar levels to stabilize, to allow your energy and appetite for good foods to return. Ask yourself, Does nibbling a little bit of sweets lead to eating a lot? Does a "the more I have, the more I want" syndrome kick in when you eat something sweet? If the answer is yes, don't set sugar up as a forbidden fruit. This gives sweets a seductive attractiveness that adds to their magnetism for people who feel like rebelling. What's forbidden is especially sweet. The coupling of guilt with pleasure often sets the trap in place. Rather acknowledge that you are making the choice not to allow *any* food to take power over you. If it would help, memorize 1 Corinthians 6:12.

No food tastes good enough and provides enough joy to rob you of your freedom and well-being!

As you become aware of (and possibly alarmed at) your intake of sugar, be careful not to replace it with artificial sweeteners. As long as you continue to use either sugar-laden foods *or* sugar substitutes, you will keep your taste buds alive for sugar. Your goal is to cut back on its use, so that you reduce your need to have *everything* taste sweet.

As you allow your taste buds to change, you'll be able to meet your desire for sweetness in a safer way. Try fruits and other naturally sweet foods—God's provision for our inborn preference for sweets.

Remember also that there are no guarantees for the safety of chemicals, be it saccharin or aspartame or any new one to come. The final word on their effects will not be in for years. As bad as sugar may be, and whatever the health hazards associated with its overuse, at least it's not chemical. It has been used for centuries.

When in doubt, leave it out!

Salt: don't pass it! "Please pass the salt." What an *overused* phrase. It's time to shake the habit. The taste for salt is conditioned; as you use less of it, your tastes change so that you begin to enjoy foods without it. Be patient with yourself and your family, but gradually cut back the use of salt in cooking and eliminate snacks that are *triple threats:* high in salt, fat and calories.

Salt's chemical name is sodium chloride, with sodium being the primary health concern. Everyone requires some sodium, but there's more than enough naturally present in foods to supply this requirement. Most Americans consume five to twenty-five times more sodium than they need.

Excessive consumption of sodium is a contributing factor in many diseases, the most prevalent being hypertension and kidney disease. Excess salt causes temporary build-up of body fluids in your system. This forces your heart to work harder to pump blood through the cardiovascular system, potentially causing high blood pressure. I do not encourage my clients to attempt to cut out salt entirely, but to cut back on its overuse.

An ounce of prevention is worth a pound of cure. Identify sources of sodium in your diet, and accept the challenge of learning to cook and enjoy foods without added fat and salt!

How Do I
Shake the Salt Habit?

- Cut back on highly processed foods and salty

snacks. This will reduce your sodium intake substantially.

- Leave the salt shaker off the table. This will help break the salt-before-you-taste habit. You'll quickly begin to enjoy the natural flavors of foods without covering them with salt. Try substituting herbs and spices for some of the salt.
- Add herb blends rather than salt to dishes. Use one of the wonderful salt-free blends from your grocer or try making your own. Keep the herb blends in a large-holed shaker right by the stove where the salt used to be. You can automatically cut a recipe's salt amount by one-half. If you substitute herbs, you can cut the salt down to one-fourth.

Seasoning Blend I

2 tsp. dry mustard	1 tsp. garlic powder
1-1/2 tsp. oregano	1 tsp. curry powder
1 tsp. marjoram	1/2 tsp. onion powder
1 tsp. thyme	1/2 tsp. celery seed

Seasoning Blend II

1 tbsp. garlic powder	1-1/2 tsp. pepper
1 tbsp. dry mustard	1 tsp. basil
1 tbsp. paprika	1/2 tsp. thyme

Watch Out for These High-Sodium Foods

- Any pickled or brine-cured food, such as sauerkraut, pickles and olives.
- Any salt-cured or smoked food, such as ham, bacon and sausage.
- Any cold cut, such as bologna, hot dogs, pastrami

and salami.

- Condiments, such as soy sauce, ketchup and chili sauce. Use in moderation.
- Convenience foods, such as canned vegetables and soups and frozen meals.

Breaking the caffeine habit. A relatively mild stimulant, caffeine is among the world's most widely used and addictive drugs. Ironically, caffeine remains an acceptable way of artificially stimulating the brain at a time when society is being exhorted to "just say no." Caffeine works by blocking one of the brain's natural sedatives, a chemical called adenosine. It stimulates the central nervous system and can elevate the mood. But, like other drugs, there is a downside to caffeine; even small amounts of it may cause side effects, including restlessness and disturbed sleep, heart palpitations, stomach irritation, fibrocystic breast disease and diarrhea. It can promote irritability, anxiety and mood disturbances. Caffeine can also aggravate PMS in women.

The stimulant effect is thought to kick in with consumption of some 150 to 250 milligrams of caffeine—the amount in one to two cups of brewed coffee or three glasses of iced tea. It adds up quickly. I encourage my patients to cut back caffeine consumption to this amount. If, after cutting back to this amount, they continue to have side effects, I encourage them to withdraw altogether.

Be careful though; in many people caffeine withdrawal causes a zombie-like fatigue and headaches and may last for up to five days. Set a goal and cut back slowly.

Brenda always comes to my mind in discussions about caffeine's "withdrawal" effects. Brenda certainly drank more coffee than most, upwards of three to four *pots* a day. When

87

she went to stay with friends one weekend, she did not realize they had recently switched to decaffeinated coffee, and they did not think to mention it. She drank a characteristic ten to twelve cups of coffee that first evening, not realizing it was all decaffeinated. She awakened Saturday morning violently ill, shaky and sluggish with a painful headache. She stayed in bed all day and evening. When she awakened on Sunday still very sick, Brenda's friend mentioned she may just need a "real" cup of coffee. A shocked Brenda found that it took only two strong cups of caffeinated coffee to cure her—of her withdrawal sickness! This experience of withdrawal was intense enough to speak to Brenda and her friends about the drug caffeine really is. She finally made the switch to decaffeinated but did so very s-l-o-w-l-y.

Eating small, balanced meals throughout the day reduced her reliance on caffeine for energy. It will work for you too. *You can say good-bye to being a caffeine junkie.*

There are five major sources of caffeine.

Coffee. The amount of caffeine in coffee depends on a number of factors: how it's brewed and for how long; whether it's regular-ground or instant. Brewed, ground coffee contains the highest level of caffeine, packing eighty-five milligrams per cup. Instant coffee is slightly lower, containing sixty milligrams per cup. This is not enough of a difference to choose instant coffee as the best choice; the goal is to reduce your intake of either. Decaffeinated brands have just a few milligrams of caffeine per cup. Many "withdrawers" do well to come off slowly by mixing decaffeinated beans with caffeinated (half and half) as their body adjusts. Be sure to look for naturally decaffeinated (Swiss Water Process) coffees, which are decaffeinated without chemicals.

Tea. A cup of brewed tea will typically have about one-third the caffeine of a cup of noninstant coffee; the longer it brews, the higher the caffeine level. A number of decaffeinated teas are available.

Sodas. Generally, the cola beverages have the highest levels of caffeine (thirty-six to fifty milligrams per serving), but look at the labels, as some fruit-flavored sodas contain caffeine. Some, including Mountain Dew and Dr. Pepper, contain almost as much as coffee or tea. This is a matter of great concern for children. Two or more such beverages are equivalent in the body of a 60-pound child to the caffeine in eight cups of coffee for a 175-pound man. Of course the problems with soda are bigger than the caffeine. Most sodas contain ten to twelve teaspoons of sugar per can; the diet sodas just replace the sugar with chemicals.

Chocolate. Cocoa beans contain caffeine, so any chocolate is suspect. The caffeine in a cup of hot chocolate is usually one-half the amount in a cup of brewed coffee (fifty milligrams). One ounce of baking chocolate contains about one-third the caffeine of a cup of coffee.

Over-the-counter drugs. Read labels carefully! Stimulants such as No-Doz and Vivarin as well as many diet pills, decongestants and headache pills supply as much caffeine as two cups of regular brewed coffee.

X
Thou Shalt
Never Go on a Fad Diet

I consider the word *diet* to be a four-letter word. It speaks defeat and depression and means *temporary*. We go *on* diets only to go *off* them. We are "good" only to be "bad." We are "legal" and then we "cheat." You don't need to set yourself up for a starvation-gorge way of existence while your weight goes up and down like a yo-yo. You don't need to look at weight loss as a punishment of eating awful-tasting and worse-looking foods or of swallowing pills, potions or supplements. A lifetime way of eating cannot exclude any major food group or nutrient, nor will it claim any food to be "magic."

Dieting always begins with firm resolve and white-knuckle discipline—until the pain of living without food becomes unbearable. As magical as they may seem, there are *no* quick-fix ways of losing weight and maintaining your health. You likely knew that before you bought this book. But it's a lot easier to diet than to change eating habits. We Americans will buy anything and drink anything if we think it will make us lose weight. There are millions to be made by marketers willing to take advantage of our obsession with the scale and dieting, and the market is unending, as more than 95 percent of the people who go on fad, quick-fix diets within a year regain the weight lost.

The dieting dilemma. Understand that the human body is "fearfully and wonderfully made" (see Ps. 139:14). Our early ancestors were subject to the ups and downs of feast and famine; only those who could maintain a steady weight could survive. You see, the body was created with "fat cells" for storing food energy for emergencies—famine.

A human baby produces a certain number of fat cells, depending upon genetics and how he or she is fed. The baby never loses these cells, and the body can add more if over-fed for an extended period of time.

It appears that the more fat cells we have, the hungrier we feel; they are continually signaling the brain to feed them.

If we drastically cut our food intake by going on a fad or self-imposed diet, our bodies will slip into a starvation mode. Our metabolism will slow down, using fewer calories than usual. And to make matters worse when we're wanting to lose weight, each fat cell appears to have a built-in "gauge"—which tries to maintain in itself a certain amount of fat.

This is the reason for plateaus in dieting (which will occur even in balanced, sensible weight loss). The body recognizes a certain weight it has been before by the amount of fat in the fat cells, and it will do everything it can to maintain that level. In a plateau the body will attempt to slow down metabolically, hold fluid and even increase the appetite, all attempts to maintain the body's weight. In healthy weight loss the plateau will be broken in three or four weeks; the body releases the "gauge." But when the diet is an unbalanced, unhealthy one, the body holds on to its weight even more stubbornly and will regain what is finally lost even more quickly. You don't have to go back to gorging to gain back your weight lost with a fad diet; your body does it for you.

You will not so easily fall into this trap if you follow the healthy pattern of eating I've outlined here in the Ten Commandments of Good Nutrition. You will be feeding your body in such a way that it will best deal with the symptoms of plateau action. The metabolism may start to slow, but your even eating throughout the day will help to keep it burning relatively high. Your body's blood sugars may fluctuate to increase your appetite, but your balanced, frequent eating will hold them stable. Your body may retain fluid, but your new healthy way of eating and drinking water will force the fluids to be released. Most important, you are not starving the body, setting yourself up for an eventual gorge. You are learning a fabulous lifetime pattern of eating and living. *Eating to lose weight is a lot more fun than starving.*

Fad fallacies. All fad diets are variations on four themes (or schemes) of deception: fasting or semistarvation (fewer than six hundred calories per day); the food-combining diet;

the high-carbohydrate, low-protein diet; and the high-protein, low-carbohydrate diet. Let's look at each. How do they work?

Fasting or semistarvation. Going without all food for weight loss can be just as drastic for the overweight person as binging. It is extreme and extremely unhealthy. If you are going to fast, make sure you are doing so for the pure purpose of prayer and intercession—in the light of God's grace. Do not fast with the impure, improper motive of weight loss, "cleansing your body" or paying "penance" for overeating.

Starving your body will certainly prompt weight loss, but, as seen in Nazi concentration camps, what you lose is primarily water and muscle weight. This may look great on the scale, but *terrible* on your body. To make matters worse, you so slow down the body's metabolism that it takes up to a year for it to normalize. This is why you gain back the weight so quickly. After starvation a return to even normal eating (not the usual binge) will cause your body to store the calories as fat. What comes off will come back on—and on—and on!

The food-combining diet. This type of diet typically has you eating protein just one time a day, robbing the body of its valuable functions. Again, if you do not balance your intake of carbohydrate and protein, your body cannot use the protein you do eat in an optimal body-building way. Your body cannot store protein throughout a day. It's a use-it-or-lose-it nutrient.

In this diet you will lose weight—along with your protein nourishment, immunities and well-being. Many people on this type of plan become anemic and protein malnourished, all in the name of health.

The high-carbohydrate, low-protein diet. This type of diet so robs your body of essential protein that it throws off your fluid balance and dehydrates your body. It appeals to your body's desire for carbohydrates (usually deprived in the typical fad diet), but it deprives your body just the same. You can lose weight quickly on a protein-deficient diet, but the initial loss is just water weight. Continued use of this low-protein diet will tear down your muscle mass; the body must have protein to repair and rebuild from normal wear and tear on the body.

The high-protein, low-carbohydrate diet. This type of fad diet has turned America against energy-giving carbohydrates with the lie that they make us fat. This diet can come packaged in a book with a lot of hype and promotion or in a formula to mix up; freeze-dried or in prepackaged meals. But it will totally unbalance your body and its fluids. Remember that carbohydrate is *the* energy fuel for your body; it spares protein from being used as energy.

From a pear to a pumpkin. If you stay on these unhealthy diets for more than two weeks, you will lose more than water weight and more than you bargained for: You begin to lose your muscle mass. And because muscle mass weighs more than fat, you will lose quickly on the scale (translated as *success*). Sadly, the weight you gain back (and you always do) is *fat* (translated as *failure*).

Years of this kind of dieting will leave you in terrible shape. Losing muscle weight only to gain back fat causes you to go from a larger pear shape to a smaller pear shape, back to a larger pear shape, down to a smaller pear shape, until you deposit the regained fat in new places and finally grow into a pumpkin shape!

This had happened to Katie, the client I introduced to you in chapter 1. By the time Katie had come to see me, not only did she weigh more than she ever had, she was "fatter" than she had ever been. Years of going up and down the scale with yo-yo dieting had changed Katie's fat deposits (research confirms this to happen), and she had begun to gain in new places. Like many women, Katie had always struggled with excess weight in the hips and thighs, but in recent years it had become more and more difficult to lose in those areas. Each time she lost then regained weight, the fat deposited through the abdominal area and her arms. It gave her that "pumpkin-shaped" feeling—and look!

The only desirable way to lose fat is through a leaning-down process that comes from a balanced intake of nutrients. On an unbalanced diet, you lose your money, your energy and your health—a risk not worth taking.

It's time to break the diet mentality with a nutritional plan that works for life. You *can* feel better, have abundant energy from morning till night and look radiant and healthy. You *can* change. With your new life-style of healthy eating, wellness is a giant step closer!

The Ten Commandments of Good Nutrition

I. Thou shalt always eat a protein with a carbohydrate (and vice versa).

II. Thou shalt never skip breakfast.

III. Thou shalt eat a healthy meal or healthy snack every three to four hours and have your healthy snack handy.

IV. Thou shalt double your fiber.

V. Thou shalt believe your mother was right: Eat your fruits and veggies.

VI. Thou shalt get your vitamins and minerals

from food, not pills.

VII. Thou shalt drink at least eight glasses of water a day.

VIII. Thou shalt trim the fat from your diet.

IX. Thou shalt consume a minimum of sugar, salt and caffeine.

X. Thou shalt never, never go on a fad diet.

SEVEN

STRESS: YOU CAN CUT ITS COST

Just as your body is designed to work for you nutritionally, it is designed to survive the stresses of life. But again most of us don't know how to make our bodies work for us when it comes to handling stress.

No one needs a definition for *stress*. Most of us are experienced experts. But stress is triggered by different things in different people. What is challenging to you may be incredibly stressful to me.

Some days we face intense crisis-oriented stress. Some people live a level of day-to-day stress that makes them feel chronically out of control to one degree or another. This chronic type of stress takes a particular toll on the body, because, though it fluctuates, it never really goes away. Although we wait to get through this stress this month or this week, there is always another stressful situation waiting for us. I've heard people joke that things don't get better—or worse—they just get different.

We humans respond to stress spiritually, emotionally and physically. And our emotional and spiritual reactions can depend on the emotional and spiritual atmospheres we live in. If our emotions are thriving on love and nurturance, stress can stretch us into new and healthy places. If our spirits are thriving on faith, stress can push us to new growth and renewed vision.

Our physical response to stress is more universal, as it is set by an elaborate, innate programming. We were created to survive, and our bodies are finely tuned to adapt to ensure that we do.

Fight or Flight

We respond to stress with a "fight or flight" mechanism that works like this: Our bodies recognize stress as danger—as if a grizzly bear had stepped across our path. We were created to survive by responding in one of two ways: by running away— flight—or by fighting this dangerous bear. To allow us optimum defense, the brain secretes chemicals that tell the body to go into a conservation mode. This state of conservation includes three predictable physical reactions that clearly affect our weight, appetite and mood.

The body's metabolism slows, storing excess energy for the fight or flight. The metabolic slow-down explains a portion of the quick weight gain that accompanies stressful times. Whether or not we eat more when under stress, the stressed body does more damage with what comes in than a nonstressed body.

The body's blood sugar dips, stimulating an appetite for high-calorie foods that will provide needed energy. As the blood sugars fluctuate, energy drops, moods drop, but appetite soars. Yes, there's a physical reason for getting tired and cranky in stressful times. And, yes, there's a physical reason for craving M&M's. (Compound this with emotions asking for food to tranquilize the anxiety, and iron-will discipline crumbles.) You may notice that *stressed* spelled backward is *desserts!*

The body retains excess fluids, keeping the systems "lubricated" for the defense. The extra fluid leads to a bloated, sluggish feeling.

The stress chemicals also affect the GI tract, often causing irritation, constipation or diarrhea.

Because our modern-day stress is not prompted by a grizzly bear, we generally do not experience the resolution or release that comes with either the fight or the flight. Because we have to "grin and bear it" rather than fight it or protest in a healthy way, our bodies stay in the stress response with all its accompanying symptoms. (Interestingly, research shows that the body's physical response to both positive and negative stress appears to be the same; the body can't discern the difference!)

The Nutritional Strategy

Never is there a more important time for good nutrition than when we are under stress. But in those stressful times we become most easily distracted from wellness principles.

A strategy of good nutrition can provide a deflective shield against the physical symptoms of stress. As the body's metabolism slows, properly timed and balanced eating can gear it up. As the blood sugars fluctuate, the right foods at the right time can undergird them, keeping them even and high. As the body retains more fluids, adequate protein and fluid intake helps restore proper fluid balance

Exercise: Your Ticket to Stress Release

As vital as good nutrition is to total wellness, it is only one of the spokes in the wellness wheel. The proper combination of balanced eating and balanced exercise is an unbeatable way to total well-being; it is the combination for living well! If stress is a way of life for you, this dynamic duo is your shield and sword to overcome your body's physical response. They are the *stress busters*.

Good nutrition can serve as a *defensive* shield, deflecting the symptoms of stress, and exercise is the *offensive* tool— the sword in your hand—that can cut off the stress responses that were never meant to be chronically activated.

Some people exercise to burn a few calories. Some exercise to reap its cardiovascular-strengthening benefits. But when you choose exercise as a life-style, you are protecting your body from the negative effects of prolonged stress.

As I have said, when sensing danger, the brain secretes chemicals that tell the body to fight or flee, setting in motion the symptoms of stress, from a slowed metabolism to gastrointestinal distress. But aerobic exercise, simulating the physical exertion inherent in the "fight" or "flight," prompts the release of stress-busting chemicals called endorphins. Working somewhat like morphine, endorphins tell the body that it is no longer in danger. (You killed or outran the grizzly.) You took control of the stressful situation; it no longer controls you.

Pete may portray for you this valuable aspect of exercise. He had overcome many entrapping behaviors with his change in eating. By eating right things at the right time, he could defensively deal with the symptoms of stress in his life. By undergirding his blood sugar fluctuations with properly timed and balanced eating, his energy stayed at a high, even keel and kept his body actively metabolizing the nutrients he was eating. But when his business stress moved to a higher level of intensity, his positive eating patterns alone could not support the stress demands.

Exercise was the key for Pete to "ride the wave" of stress rather than getting caught in its undertow. In the past, when things would get stressful, the time and energy expended in exercise were just too costly; it was the first activity to be cut. But now, armed with knowledge and a new perspective on exercise, he starts his day with hard, brisk walking as his offensive tool to cut off his body's stress response. It has become his way to cut the costs of stress.

People frequently ask how often they need to exercise. The answer always depends upon the individual's goals. A person actively seeking fitness needs to exercise four or five times each week. A person working to maintain good fitness should exercise three or four times each week. A person under intensive stress may need some form of exercise every day, as it is *the* physical way to process that stress effectively. When our lives are most stressful—when we have the *least amount of time* to exercise—we have the most to gain from it.

What Does Exercise Do for You?

- Exercise increases metabolism and decreases appetite.
- Exercise is great not only for the body, but also for the mind. It increases self-esteem, improves general appearance and gives you a wonderful sense of well-being!
- Aerobic exercise increases your protection against heart disease by improving your heart's condition (making it more efficient) and increasing your

HDL cholesterol (the good guy!). Any exercise that raises your pulse to a training rate or, more simply, gets you breathing hard is an aerobic exercise. The benefits occur from achieving that increased pulse rate and maintaining it for at least twenty straight minutes three times a week. Most exercise experts encourage gradually increasing your exercise time up to an hour every other day.

- Exercise breaks the plateaus or "set points" of weight loss. It is an external way of boosting the metabolism naturally lowered in the body's attempt to maintain a certain weight.

- Remember, exercise is nature's best tranquilizer. Just thirty minutes of aerobic exercise a day is one of the tried and true methods of releasing tension. Exercise is *the* healthy outlet for the stress of the world, certainly a more acceptable alternative than eating, drinking or smoking!

- Recent studies have shown that exercise seems to be a vital factor in promoting excellent bone growth and life-long maintenance. A well-planned exercise routine may stimulate the development of strong bone mass and later slow down any bone loss occurring as a result of osteoporosis. Exercise increases the circulation and flow of nutrients to the bone, encouraging new bone growth and building. Without routine exercise bones may shrink, weaken and become porous.

  The best exercises to build strong bones are the weight-bearing type, such as brisk walking, jumping rope and bicycling. As bones are stressed from these activities, they become stronger and denser. Swimming, although an excellent aerobic exercise,

is not as effective in strengthening bones. To prevent and reduce the effects of osteoporosis, it is
recommended that one exercise at least every other
day for twenty-five to thirty minutes.

Exercising for Life!

You can't store fitness. Consistent exercise will help you
have more energy, better concentration, less depression,
better sleep and ammunition against disease. You will have
improved wellness, physically and emotionally. Commitment
to an exercise routine that goes hand-in-hand with good nutrition is one of the greatest gifts you can ever give yourself.

Despite the benefits of exercise, it is nonetheless difficult
to find a program you can stick to and enjoy. Consequently,
many people have a history of start-and-stop exercising.
Others consistently drive themselves to work out, but derive
little pleasure from it. Still others simply avoid exercise
altogether. If you fall into one of these categories, odds are
that you haven't found the exercise pattern that's right for
you. To jump on the fitness bandwagon—and stay on it—
you need to select an exercise that matches your life-style
and fills your physical needs.

The major aerobic activities are brisk walking, running,
swimming and bicycling. Aerobic dance combines the toning
benefits of calisthenics with a good heart workout and stress
release. You can find a number of routines to fit your needs,
but you're apt to stick with the ones that you find the most fun.

Brisk walking works the very best for me. I can walk in
my neighborhood or anywhere business takes me. I can walk
at the time of day that best fits my schedule and when the
weather best suits a walk. I have periodically tried other forms
of exercise (aerobics classes, racquetball and health clubs,

and I ran for many years), but walking is the form that fits me best. When our schedule permits, my husband and I walk together, often in silence just enjoying exercising and the time together. I also enjoy walking alone; it is my time to be outside, seeing and experiencing the world God has created. It is my time to "divert daily" from the demands and stresses of life and to walk and talk with God.

The exercises you'll find most enjoyable will probably be those you feel you can best handle. If you have difficulty with eye-hand coordination, for example, you may be frustrated by a sport like tennis but do well with walking or swimming. If you are not naturally flexible, you may be happier with bicycling than ballet.

Consider the shape you are in. If you are overweight, any activity that involves pounding on your feet, such as running or aerobic dance, may stress your joints by placing too much weight on them. Try riding a stationary bike or swimming instead.

If you're over thirty-five, most exercise experts encourage you to see a health professional for an "all-points" check before beginning an exercise program.

I advise newcomers to regular exercise to consider walking—an excellent beginning exercise. Measure off a mile and walk it briskly. How long did it take you to walk that mile? Gradually increase your pace, so you are walking it in fifteen minutes. Now add a second mile and work up to a pace of two miles in thirty minutes. Then add a third mile and work till you can walk the three miles in forty to forty-five minutes. By starting with something you already can do—and do anytime, anywhere—you'll be more amenable to building it up into a regular routine.

Think of exercise as an act of kindness to your body, not a punishment. Start slowly and avoid overtaxing yourself.

The biggest mistake people make is doing too much, too soon. Set realistic goals.

Be sure to warm up before exercise and cool down afterward. By warming up your muscles—stretching them, then beginning your exercise at a slow pace—you help prevent injury. Cooling down—exercising at a slower pace, then finally stretching the muscles—helps stop them from tightening up and cramping.

I know some people who feel there is no enjoyable form of exercise. If you're one of them, remind yourself that exercise can be a "sword in your hand"—cutting off the stress mechanism and lowering your level of stress. Who could give up such an opportunity?

Remember, exercise is a vital tool for fighting chronic stress and keeping your body fit and working for you. Let it be something you are choosing to do—for life!

EIGHT

PHYSICAL CHANGE: THE CHALLENGES

As you embark on a plan based on the Ten Commandments of Good Nutrition, you can expect to face physiological and emotional adjustments to the change. It will take at least five to six days before the change begins to feel physically comfortable. You can expect the following:

First and second days: You will feel slightly sluggish, irritable and dissatisfied with your eating.

Third day: This will be one of your most difficult days as your body will begin to feel the chemical change. It may seem that every cell in your body is crying out for food, particularly something sweet. Expect this day to be a struggle, but not an impossible one to overcome.

Fourth day: If you make it through the third day without overeating, this one won't be so difficult.

Fifth day: This is the day of the ravenous appetite; you

can expect to be *hungry* for food, not sweets necessarily, just *food*. You can eat a meal and still have the feeling: That was a good appetizer. What else is there to eat?

Sixth and seventh days: By now it is getting easier and easier; you have more energy, and you have more control over your appetite. You are on the road to a lifetime of good eating.

Remember, the third and fifth days are always the most difficult. Circle them on your calendar in red!

I know this sounds more like a withdrawal from a strongly addictive drug than simply allowing your body to adjust to a wonderfully healthy way of eating. But let's face reality: Putting *in* the healthy foods means leaving *out* the unhealthy, and that means a chemical change—a withdrawal of sorts. I would prefer you know what to expect than to give up in defeat as soon as you get started.

Remember Katie—despairing on her first visit to me? Right then and there, we developed a new plan of eating for her, based on the principles of the Ten Commandments of Good Nutrition and designed to meet her own needs best. As I advised Katie as to what to expect in the days ahead, we discussed these chemical changes and adjustments of her body. She quickly saw that "chemistry" was the culprit of her many false-start attempts at dieting. Every Monday morning was the same for Katie: She would awaken filled with motivation to "get back on her diet" or to start a new one. Every Monday afternoon was also the same for Katie: She would "hit the wall" at 3:30 or so and fall into forbidden food. Even if she was able to make it through Monday with a firm resolve of willpower, that too would crumble when Wednesday's withdrawal pains began. By the time Friday's hungries hit, she knew the weekend was here, so why get started again until Monday? Katie repeated the pattern week after week after week.

If, like Katie, you have been living out this weekly pattern of defeat, you most likely soothed the withdrawal pains with food. This time Katie realized that it was a necessary (but temporary!) part of breaking free into a lifetime of good eating. She was able to speak back to the appetite and hunger, choosing instead to eat nourishing, healthy foods. By the sixth day her energy and appetite began to stabilize, and the surprise of feeling good made it all worth the effort. She could see that it was possible.

Cravings: Real or Imagined?

Even after you have physically adjusted to the new way of eating, you will sometimes crave certain unhealthy foods you "used to love." You miss that old favorite!

These cravings can be the undoing of your freedom. When you feel you are craving a particular food, evaluate your day. Did you get off your routine of eating the right foods at the right time? Did you go too long without a meal or snack? Did you miss out on proper balance of carbohydrates and proteins? If so, the physical you is sending out a message. It's saying, "Feed me! I *need* food!"

The best way to handle cravings is to try to prevent them. Resist getting off track and returning to sporadic, erratic eating. This is especially important when you are most stressed and most vulnerable to the emotional messages that signal you to eat. When the feelings get too hot to handle, it may seem simpler to return to the "old way of eating" than to change your way of dealing with life.

The most nutritional meal plan in the world will be of little value if left in the top drawer. It must be fit into your lifestyle, which may need to change to accommodate it. Some unhealthy eating patterns are habitual, and old habits can be triggered into action by memories, stress, even old friends.

Change: The Emotional Challenge

You have already taken the biggest step in the challenge of change: You know you need to change, and you desire to make it happen. This desire is necessary, as change is hard to face and carry through. It requires commitment and energy. Habits that have been developing for a lifetime will require patience for you to unlearn and let go.

Newness and change can be terrifying! Let yourself feel the fear of change, as *denying the threat of the new will keep you in the old*.

To make room for change, we must let go of destructive behavior patterns, leave behind self-defeating behaviors. "There is a time for everything, and a season for every activity under heaven...a time to tear down and a time to build" (Eccl. 3:1,3). There is not room within you for both old patterns and the new.

Whenever you let go of the old, you experience loss. It happens when you leave a neighborhood you know and love, when you marry or have children and lose freedom, when you change jobs, when parents die, when children leave the nest. You also experience loss when letting go of old behaviors and habits. In every transition, happy or sad, we're called to let go of what was. Until we do, we can't appreciate what is.

Facing a loss, we humans need to grieve. We need to allow ourselves to release the pain within, so we can return to a state of balance. You may feel depressed, lonely, guilty, helpless, angry, panicked, resentful, hopeless and hostile before you finally feel relief. Give yourself permission to feel all the emotions that rise to the surface as you leave behind habits that do not promote a healthy life-style. Keeping a journal can help you identify what might otherwise be vague feelings of anxiety. Look at yourself and your feelings with candor. Take time each day to reflect on your progress.

"I don't know what's wrong with me. I love the way I'm eating. I love the way I'm feeling. I'm even starting to like the way I'm looking! I have more energy than I've had since high school. I'm even starting to grow nails!" Katie was in my office six weeks after our first visit. She truly had made some amazing changes in her eating and perspectives about food. She had lost about ten pounds on the scale, although measurements of her muscle-to-fat ratio were showing she had lost even more fat. She was simultaneously replacing valuable muscle mass that had been lost through years of unhealthy eating. She did look and feel marvelous, yet something was wrong

"I was at the grocery store this morning and just started sobbing—right there in front of the breakfast cereals! There were so many to choose from, all claiming to be the best for me, and I just broke down, feeling overwhelmed. It wasn't that I was confused; I knew which to buy. I just don't know what I'm feeling. But I've been depressed all day."

I had a clue about what Katie was feeling; she was experiencing loss. She was grieving, thereby experiencing a myriad of emotions from a myriad of sources. She was sad and mad, panicked and helpless all at the same time. Katie was grieving for a lot of losses: the carefree, careless way she used to eat, the foods she used to eat, the way she *used eating*, even the weight she was losing for the last time. She was gladly giving up many of these, but she still had to let go. And that meant she had to let go of some grief as well.

Sabotage or Support?

A major challenge in your personal change will be dealing with the reactions of your family and friends. Your change is as scary to them as it is to you. They are losing a familiar you, seeing a new image of you.

Many family members want to see you lose weight and succeed as long as they can control it. If they can take the credit, they will help. But if they feel that you are doing this on your own, they often feel they have more to lose than to gain. As unhealthy as you may be in your present state, it may be comfortable for them to have you this way. This is especially true of spouses. Let's look at how husbands, and then wives, can sabotage a mate's efforts.

"I'll pay you ten dollars for every pound you lose."

"Lose twenty-five pounds in the next two months, and I'll buy you a new wardrobe."

"Get into that bathing suit, and we'll go on a cruise."

Husbands often try to motivate their wives to lose weight. But actually they are the least likely to be helpful, as they are too personally involved and too invested in success.

Most often husbands want to see their wives lose weight, but they fall short of offering positive assistance. Why? Subconsciously they may fear their wives' success, and the fear may sabotage any helpful efforts. There is so much at stake: loss of eating as a form of entertainment and a change of diet that may mean new foods are served and old ones lose their "favored food status." As a wife becomes more physically attractive, a husband may become more insecure.

The sabotage may be subtle complaints about the "new way of eating." ("Why don't we ever have anything good to eat anymore?" "This tastes awful! You used to be such a good cook!" "Well, honey, you can eat anyway you want, but don't mess with my food, because I'm not the one with the problem.")

Sometimes the sabotage is much more direct; he'll bring home ice cream or donuts or boxes of candy.

Katie had unknowingly been fighting this "submerged sabotage" for her entire married life. Although her husband, Roger, would promise her exotic vacations and wardrobes if she could just "lose this weight," she began to see that the sabotage would start a few weeks after the diet was showing success. It was very subtle. Roger would make discouraging remarks such as "You don't seem to be losing like you should. Are you sure you're not cheating?" "Are you sure that's on your diet?" "When is this diet really going to work, so I can have a pretty wife again?" A few weeks later he would bring home "surprises" of Katie's favorite eclairs, because Katie had been so good on that awful diet. Before long he was complaining to friends about how boring and tasteless Katie's cooking was now, and he had to eat out to get a decent meal. All the while Roger was holding out the promise of that new wardrobe or cruise.

Likewise, wives often sabotage their husbands' attempts to change eating patterns. They often start out being supportive: buying and cooking food in a healthier fashion. But when the husband begins to succeed in his health goals (leaning down, gaining energy, keeping an exercise regimen), things change on the homefront.

"Pam, you can't believe it! I came home last night, and Mary had baked macadamia nut, chocolate chip cookies, just for me! She said that I had lost all the weight I needed to lose, that I deserved a special treat. When I tried to say thanks, but no thanks, she blew up at me and told me she was sick of all this healthy eating, and it was time things got back to normal." Ron knew that things weren't going back to the way they used to be. He had embraced a new perspective about wellness, one that went far beyond his weight, and one that he was not about to give up. Interestingly, Mary had changed right along with Ron and honestly loved their new way of eating and thinking. But she didn't expect him to get so attractive again. She didn't feel as secure in their relationship, and she resented Ron's jokingly saying, "Mary was killing me with food!"

Mary's sabotage was a direct measure of the fear she was experiencing, similar to Katie's sabotaging husband but with an added twist: Ron's success seemed to threaten her identity as the provider of "good food." It seemed to pinpoint her previous food buying and cooking patterns as the culprit. If she could sabotage the new patterns and get things back to normal, she could reduce her anxiety.

How can you hold your own against a spouse who may not even know he or she is sabotaging your efforts? Anticipate and prepare for other people's reactions. If you can expect others' negative actions and comments, you can minimize their negative effect on you.

Katie held her own by preparing herself for Roger's comments and actions. We planned ways she could respond lovingly to Roger rather than eating to spite him. She approached this as a way of eating for the whole family, not as her "problem." Katie was writing in a journal every day, and through her writing she was able to define how she felt, then talk to Roger about it. They began counseling with a pastor from their church to learn to communicate lovingly. Most important, Katie made a decision that she was changing her eating for herself—not to get a new wardrobe, not to go on a vacation. Gaining freedom was reward enough.

Like Katie, the only person capable of gaining the freedom you desire for yourself is you. Another person may not force or prevent your changing. Another person's words and actions may have an effect on you, but ultimately it is you who decides your actions. You decide what will and won't go in your mouth.

Breaking the Power of the Scale

Breaking free out of the food trap is not just a matter of losing weight. If you have weight to lose, it comes off as a benefit of being freed from the bondage of using food as more than nourishment. Your weight on the scale is not the primary issue at stake. The issue is your eating behavior and your unhealthy relationship with food, not how many pounds you weigh.

We have used the scale as a god to tell us if we've been good or bad, if we should be happy or sad, if we can eat or have to starve today. The answers to these questions come from the one and only God who created us in His image, not from a machine that displays a deceptive number that can never, never give the whole truth. As I've pointed out, the scale has no indicator that shows how much of your weight is muscle mass, water weight or fat; it just shows a number!

If you've been a "dieter," the scale has no doubt been your license to eat. You've checked in with the scale to get quick reinforcement for your deprivation. The logic goes like this: If I'm going to give up everything I enjoy in life (my favorite foods), I surely better get a payoff! If the scale doesn't give that reward, I yell, "Not fair! If I'm not going to lose, I might as well be eating." If the scale does show a weight loss, I feel the need to celebrate how "good" I've been, and of course I celebrate with food. Then I weigh myself after the celebration; if I didn't gain, I feel as if I got away with it, which sets me up to try to "get away with it" again.

But weighing is a lying, deceptive, false god. Worshipping this false god every morning, or three times a day, is all part of the obsession with our weight and food.

This may sound drastic, but it's important. Weigh yourself right now. *Do not weigh yourself again for a month.* Trust in how you know you're eating; trust in how you feel your body is changing—not in what a deceptive scale can tell you. You may find that giving up this reliance on the scale is more difficult than giving up overeating. Give it a try!

This idea may make you feel threatened, even angry. We rely on that scale as if its word were God's. Of course the scale, in itself, is not an evil. But when we rely too much on those numbers, giving the scale more power than a mechanical device should have, it robs us of any peace we have at our fingertips.

You may want to close this book for a while. Spend a few days observing your eating, how your body responds and the magnetism of the scale. Then come back to these pages. Has your perspective changed? Do you see that the scale holds unhealthy power in your life? Can you trust in God rather than the scale god? This lesson and discipline may be difficult, but it will be important for you to examine before you read part 3.

LIFE (Living In Freedom Everyday)

Freedom over food has to include freedom from the scale and freedom from dieting. Obsessive, unhealthy, deprived *dieting* is not any more of a freedom than obsessive, unhealthy *overeating*. Being physically free over food begins by choosing a way of eating and living that is so comfortable that you can live with it the rest of your life.

Recovery begins by choosing a plan of eating that enables you to operate from a point of strength physically, a nutrition plan for life. Once you've started on that plan, you have room to look at your emotional needs and meet them appropriately.

You may say, "But this will take too long! I want to be thin now!" Well, the truth is, this *will* take longer, but the results will last. You won't be fighting the same battles day after day, month after month, year after year. You won't even be *able* to eat the same way anymore; you'll be too aware of what you're doing to your body. You will be free!

As you set out on this nutritional plan, the process you have used to achieve this goal—your new way of eating— now must become the goal. Attaining freedom is only part of the physical goal; maintaining that freedom is *the* goal.

If you aren't feeling so free, you can at least be feeling pleased with the progress you have made, feeling good about the changes in your body and your appetite. If you are feeling much more in charge, yet are still struggling with desires for food and overeating, it's time to move on.

PART III:

FREE AT LAST

NINE

LOOKING BACK

Once you see a lamp of hope shining on the physical you, it may be time to look to the *emotional you* and evaluate the roots of your unhealthy relationship with food. *Are you eating to deal with what's eating you?* Are you using food to cope with life? Your emotional needs can be met in legitimate ways—not through the use and abuse of food.

Katie: Gaining Control

Two months after her first visit to me, Katie had made many changes. She was eating in a more even and balanced way than she had in her entire life. She had lost thirteen pounds, as a side benefit of her change in eating. She had started walking most afternoons as a powerful stress release. Amazingly, she had lost thirteen pounds of fat—not lean muscle, not water and not by starving. Katie was seeing her desires for food change, now desiring foods that would benefit, not harm, her body. Yet she would occasionally let her eating habits slip out of control. The "binge" was now on good foods, and it lacked the frenzy of previous years, but it still cropped up.

As I worked with Katie, I asked her to keep a week's diary of what she ate and when. I asked her to note what she was feeling when she overate or desired to. I was trying to get a feel for the specific feeling "triggers" that would send her into a binge.

Here's what we eventually came up with: "If I am happy, I want to eat. If I am sad, I want to eat. If I am mad, I want to eat. If I am celebrating, I want to eat. If I am grieving, I want to eat. If I am anxious, I want to eat. If I am bored, I want to eat. If I am frustrated, I want to eat. If I am hurt or feel rejected or ashamed, I do eat!"

Katie saw that if she was eating the right things at the right time she could most often choose *not* to overeat, though the *desire* was there in response to just about every emotion. Katie was most vulnerable when she felt hurt or rejected. Then and there she felt she could not control the desire; it seemed to control her.

Up until this moment of insight Katie had always claimed that she simply loved the taste of food and had a hard time giving up something that gave her so much pleasure. In reality she had an emotional relationship with food, one that had started years before when the child Katie had discovered that eating certain foods made her feel better; eating a lot of certain foods made her feel a lot better!

To make permanent changes, ones that would stand up under stress, Katie had to go back and face the pain of her childhood, which she had dealt with in unhealthy ways; this pain had been the foundation for her relationship with food. In the midst of a chaotic family life Katie had used food to dull the senses and relieve the stress. To detach from food emotionally, this dependence had to be broken. The broken foundation blocks had to be repaired.

The Submerged Emerges

As you get your body into the pattern spelled out in the "Ten Commandments," it's likely that the emotions that food has helped you *submerge* will *emerge*. New feelings will bubble to the surface. If they are not pleasant, take heart! What you feel can be healed. As long as you are covering up your feelings with food, there's not a chance for healing. Once you begin to feel, your mind is being renewed. You're recovering. I wish I could say this part is easy, but it may be the hardest thing you've ever undertaken.

Denial is a formidable and deceptive tool for survival. And it is like an onion in that it is many layered. How easy it is to fill our lives to overflowing with activities, staying so busy that we can ignore—and deny—our true feelings. How many people do you know who seem to have arranged their lives so that they are "human doings" rather than "human beings"? A human doing is too busy to feel anything.

We have all developed a faulty system in one way or another. It is part of humanity; we were born into the lie. It is the same lie that Satan used on Eve in the garden (see Gen. 3:1-6). The Lie: 1) God cannot or will not meet your needs. 2) If you get your needs met in an unhealthy way or, as in the case of Adam and Eve, a sinful way, you won't experience any negative consequences. 3) You need to be your own god. If you're going to get your needs met, you'd better develop your own system for getting them met.

As you continue to read, ask the Holy Spirit to show

you which—if any—patterns have influenced your coping mechanisms.

How do you hear the Lord's voice? You ask and you listen. Don't listen for an audible voice but listen for a voice deep within your spirit. As you listen, turn also to God's Word—the first word in all we think, say and do. Look there for confirmation of the Holy Spirit's word to your spirit.

"Dear friend, I pray that you may enjoy good health and that all may go well with you, even as your soul is getting along well" (3 John 2).

Failure to Thrive

No one would argue that there is an intricate design for our physical growth. No one is born "grown up"! We come into this world as a tiny infant programmed for growth—if we are nourished with food and water. To thrive, the human body requires certain nutrients; without them, we become malnourished. A child starved of these essential nutrients will not grow properly. Medically, this is diagnosed as a "failure to thrive."

There is a similar design for a person's emotional growth. At birth we are emotionally immature, and we grow emotionally much as we grow physically. If we are deprived of our emotional "nutrients," our emotional growth is arrested. We fail to thrive. Even though the body may grow to physical maturity, the emotions can remain stunted and childlike.

As adults, we may appear to be coping with day-to-day life. But, underneath, the child in us may suffer from an overwhelming sense of shame or guilt, from self-denial, from distrust or from too much responsibility—that is, taking on the burden of something that is not ours to own.

Let's look at the childhood patterns which can cause these

misplaced emotions that become a barrier that grows into gigantic proportions.

The Family System: The Origin of the Food Trap

The versions are varied, yet time after time I see that people get caught in the food trap at a young age, when families do not properly meet their needs.

If I could describe a perfect family, it would be one that set boundaries to live by; but at the same time specific rules would be open for discussion and flexible, depending on circumstances. Each family member would have the right to express thoughts and feelings even when other family members didn't agree. A disagreement about rules wouldn't necessarily mean the rules would change, but the disagreeing family member would continue to be respected and accepted.

In a healthy family no member's needs are valued as more important than anyone else's. In this kind of family system a child has the chance to develop a sense of identity, has self-esteem and feels that personal thoughts and feelings are accepted. This child grows up able to express feelings freely and openly but chooses to do so with consideration for others.

In children emotional seeds are planted, seeds that grow as the child grows. In a healthy family system these seeds are seeds of love, respect and independence.

Not all family systems plant such healthful seeds, and these families are often called dysfunctional.

The concept of the dysfunctional family was first discussed in cases where a parent was an alcoholic. But the unhealthy relationships that characterize a dysfunctional unit are now recognized to be more universal. Even if there is no chemical dependency, an entire family can operate under the "rules" that govern an alcoholic family. These families produce *adult children* with dysfunctions and dependencies of their own.

Actually, according to John and Linda Friel in *Adult Children: The Secrets of Dysfunctional Families*, 90-95 percent of today's families are considered at least mildly dysfunctional: Family members are inflexible and can't tolerate change or conflict. Reasons behind the dysfunctional system may vary. The family may be ashamed of and trying to hide a secret or illness. To meet the expectations of their social grouping, the family may have an oppressive set of rules for behavior. The family may be striving to meet an external standard of perfection.

Whatever the reason, this dysfunctional family is not a wonderful unit in which to grow up. Members aren't allowed to question the family rules or to voice thoughts or feelings that conflict with these rules. Disagreement is met with rejection. Children from this type of home don't learn to communicate openly and directly. They don't learn that one can disagree with someone else and still have that person's respect and acceptance. Children from this sort of family don't learn who they are, what they really like and don't like or how to get their needs met.

Katie's life was the direct result of the seeds that had been planted in it. The child Katie never learned to *own*, or certainly value, her feelings. If Katie said she was cold, her mom would say, "You couldn't be. It's burning up in this house." If Katie said she was hungry, her mom would say, "You couldn't be. We just finished lunch." If Katie said she wasn't hungry, her mom would say, "Of course you are; it's dinnertime." Katie learned early on that disagreeing with her mother's I-know-what-you-need-better-than-you-do methods only caused conflict. She came to believe that she was a bad child for even thinking, much less feeling, differently. This grew into a deep sense of shame. Her thoughts weren't valuable; her feelings weren't valuable; so she was not valuable.

The emotional seeds sown in the dysfunctional family are seeds of guilt, fear and obligation; they are sown into a *soil of shame*. As children from these families grow into adulthood, these seeds grow into invisible weeds that choke out self-confidence and self-esteem. Katie had to learn to identify these weeds and how to uproot them.

Codependency and Eating Dependency: A Family System

Much has been written in recent years about the subject of codependency and its effect on families. In her book *Codependent No More*, Melody Beattie gives this definition: Codependency occurs when a person lets someone else's behavior affect him or her and becomes obsessed with controlling that behavior. Codependent people are so absorbed in other people's problems that they don't have time to identify or solve their own problems.

The dysfunctional family is often built as a codependent family system based on an unbalanced relationship between spouses, both of whom may have low self-esteem. Spouses look to each other to meet their own needs, often without directly discussing their needs or even knowing what they are. One spouse takes the role of caretaker, becoming consumed with keeping the other functioning well and in control. But the caretaker is taking on more responsibility than one human can have for another.

Being unable to meet their own needs, these adults are unable to meet the needs of their children. Instead they set up an oppressive set of rules that prevent healthy expression of feelings.

The children from this family system become afraid to express themselves, until eventually they don't have a clue as to who they are or how they feel. They learn to avoid conflict at any price, to swallow "unacceptable" thoughts and feelings so as not to upset others, and to constantly fear rejection.

Jim Herrod was a man of many needs. His mother had died of tuberculosis when he was three years old. TB also took his grandfather and two sisters the same summer. He was reared by a grieving father and grandmother who were in such pain that they built an emotional brick wall to survive. Though they worked hard to meet the surviving children's physical needs, they were otherwise emotionally unavailable. Jim remembers seeing only one emotion from his father, and that was a frightening rage that would appear from nowhere and usually end with a brutal whipping for "just being in his way." Jim left home after one of these beatings, even though he was only fourteen. He lied about his age and found a job, and a wife, in a nearby city.

Mary Herrod was the oldest of nine children. She had started cooking and cleaning for the family at age seven. Mary never remembers playing with her brothers and sisters; she was too busy helping out her mother who was too busy having babies. Mary was also too busy working to think or feel; she never learned anything about emotional needs. She grew up with only one purpose in life: to meet the physical needs of others.

Mary and Jim were the "perfect" codependent couple. Jim had such low self-worth that he was like a robot. He was consumed with succeeding in life, to show the world he was really OK. Mary took on the role of Jim's caretaker, absorbed with keeping him functioning well.

The four children from this marriage all bore different manifestations of Jim and Mary's emotional vacuum. They all learned one thing about emotional needs: Swallow them! Don't rock the boat.

People learn to be caretakers or codependent long before they can rationally choose such a way of relating to the world. As children, they don't learn how to *receive* but only *how to take care of others*—how to keep Daddy from losing his temper, for example. Once a person sets up these patterns, it is difficult for him or her to relate in any other way without outside help.

But to compound the problem, caregivers tend to be friends with other caregivers, so the life-style often continues without challenge. Codependent mothers teach their children and grandchildren by role model to be codependent, so it becomes a "curse" carried from generation to generation.

Three Family Types

The authors of the book *Bulimia: A Systems Approach to Treatment* say that eating dependencies most often come out of three types of unbalanced family systems: the perfect family, the overprotective family and the chaotic family. Let's look at these types of families and the messages they send to their members.

The "perfect" family. This family places high priority on appearances—the family's reputation, identity and achievements. The family's ruling question is, What would people think? (The coveted answer is, My, don't you have well-behaved children!) It is important that no family member stand out as different from the norm. (United we stand; divided we fall.)

The perfectionistic family does not allow mistakes. From the outside looking in, this will often seem to be a very loving and caring family. Actually, the loving and caring is just covering up a rigid set of rules, many of which govern emotions—particularly the "weak" emotions. ("If you can't show a happy face, don't show any face at all." "Don't cry, or I'll give you something to cry about!") "Tapes" played in these families are performance oriented: "A job worth doing is worth doing well." "Make us proud of you!" "You are disappointing us!" "Be good!" "You are my perfect daughter/my perfect son." "Don't let us down now."

Bridgette was the oldest of four daughters. Her father was the chief executive officer for a large manufacturing firm. Their home was an even more tightly run business with impossibly high standards of perfection. "I can't expect perfection of my employees. They don't come from the same stock as my girls do," Dad would often say. The "Quest for the Best" was their family motto. And the best was what was delivered.

At eighteen Bridgette had been valedictorian of her graduating class, had been awarded scholarships at several desirable schools and was an accomplished gymnast. She set goals and achieved them. She had no concept of working *toward* a goal; she simply felt she should succeed at whatever she tried, no matter what the costs. The costs were high; her own self-worth and acceptance of herself were based totally on her performance. If she couldn't measure up, she was worthless. And she could never measure up, because the standard was always set just a little higher than where she was.

The overprotective family. This family emphasizes the need to be close. Members tend to take too much responsibility for one another, particularly one of them who has a problem. There are no boundaries in this family; everyone is community property. Slogans of this family include these: All for one and one for all. You know we'll always be there for you. No one is good enough for you. Find someone nice to take care of you. You can't trust anyone outside the family. Are they "our" type of people? No one can love you the way we do.

Members stay enmeshed within this family because they never develop an independent life of their own. Even as adults, they do not evolve unique personalities. Parents in these families work hard to be good, caring parents; they just never quite see and hear their children clearly.

They do all the "right" things but never find out how their child feels. The child says, "I'm hungry," and the parent says, "You can't be hungry; you just ate." The child says, "I'm cold," and the parent says, "Of course you're not cold; it's hot in here!" The child says, "I'm sad," and the parent says, "You can't be; you have too much to be grateful for." Parents never "retire" from being the major influence in the lives of their children.

Merritt Herrod grew up in a citrus business. Actually, it was the family business, but the business was the family. You read about her father, Jim. He was a "self-made" man, uneducated yet extremely shrewd in business dealings. He had one of the legendary climbs to success, from working in an orange-packing house to owning vast acreage of orange groves. Merritt was the third of four children and was, for all intents and purposes, invisible to the family. Her older brother, the second child, consumed any energy the family had left over from the business. His emotional problems as a child had developed into drug problems as a teen.

The Herrod family had adopted the stance that no one could be trusted outside the family; they had to depend on each other to make it through life. Merritt had no boundaries, no psychological fence to let some things into her life and keep other things out. She also had no owning of feelings, no way of recognizing or expressing her own feelings or needs; they had to be swallowed or replaced with the corporate needs of the family. Overshadowed by her brother's problem, she retreated and isolated herself. She never learned how to form relationships outside the family unit. She had learned nothing but mistrust for people. Being with people made her feel awkward and self-conscious.

The chaotic family. The rules of this family are inconsistent or nonexistent, with neither parent emotionally available to the children. A parent's absence or abuse may be physical. A child may be neglected because of alcoholism. Some parents may provide ample material things but be unavailable for or abusive to the children emotionally.

The children of a chaotic family learn not to talk, trust or feel. Because they learn to benumb their emotions, they do not "own" their own feelings or their own reality.

Standard tapes play in this family: Don't ask questions. Do what you're told. You can't trust anyone. Do as I say and not as I do. Because I said so! I wouldn't yell at you if I didn't love you. This hurts me more than it hurts you.

Dana came from a chaotic family such as this. Her grown-up assessment of her childhood is "to call my family dysfunctional would be a compliment." But her child assessment was "no one is here for me because I am not good." Dana's father was a closet alcoholic; his drinking, though never seen and never discussed, controlled the family. Her mom was consumed with Dad's "problem," consumed with keeping up a well-respected front to friends and neighbors. She learned to benumb her own feelings and work only to keep things even. "Don't upset Mommy; she's got enough problems with Daddy." "Don't upset Daddy; it'll make his 'problem' worse." She learned to smile on the outside and cry on the inside.

All of these families are the result of unhealthy rules that have been passed down from generation to generation; accompanying pain and tragedy have been a curse likewise passed down. The dysfunctional family is not a group of bad people; it is a group of people being controlled by a set of bad rules with lives built on shame.

A Word About Shame

There are three kinds of shame, and only one of them is healthy. What some would call *humility*, this healthy shame makes us aware of our wrongs and hurting of others. Humility brings us to a place where we realize our fallibility. Here we realize that we are the created, not the Creator.

A second shame I'd call *shamelessness*—a shifting of our personal shame onto others. Because of our shame, we shame others. This shame-shifting game can be treacherous, as our words can shame others, even when spoken in so-called humor.

The third kind of shame is the most damaging. Whereas shamelessness is what we do to other people, this shame is what others have done to us. It *distorts* one's identity. It does not say, "I made a mistake"; it says, "I *am* a mistake." This shame says, "I was *born* a mistake." Even with a deep faith in God, you can feel that you are different from others. Though you don't know exactly why, it's harder for God to love you than it is for Him to love other people.

What causes the distorting shame? *Words can cause shame.* They become tapes that play over and over in your mind. If you hear and believe words that are not true, they

133

can lead you down a destructive path.

There is tremendous power in words. Proverbs 18:21 tells us that death and life are in words that are spoken: "The tongue has the power of life and death." Wise Solomon knew that sticks and stones may break my bones, but words *can* hurt me—even to the point of death, killing the truth of who we have been created to be. Some examples of destructive spoken words are "You can't do anything right"; "You'll never be anything but trouble"; "You'll never amount to anything"; "If you really love us, you'll make us proud of you"; "You're going to fight with your weight all your life"; "You're so lazy...so unlovable...so dumb...so stupid...such a pig." Such horrible, shaming words, many times spoken carelessly, can control our lives.

Abandonment can cause shame. This might be physical abandonment by divorce, desertion or death of a parent. Or it could be emotional abandonment; a physically present parent can ignore a child's emotional needs. The adult child can spend a lifetime trying to fill those unmet needs. An abandoned child cannot understand why he or she has been deserted or ignored by this all-perfect parent (a child cannot picture a parent as anything less than perfect), so the child bears the responsibility for the wrongdoing, internalizing the shame built on a lie: I must be bad because I made him or her leave me.

Emotional or physical abuse can cause shame. The statistics are staggering. One out of four women have been sexually abused. One out of eight men have been abused. When the very person who is there to take care of you abuses you, you have been abandoned. The sense of shame is deep, built on a modified version of the lie mentioned above: I must be bad because I made him hurt me.

Some people cannot remember many details of their

childhood. In blocking out the intense pain, they have blocked out the whole scene. Yet the bad days are there, an emotional vacuum that is packed in shame, false guilt and a horrible distortion of self-worth.

This distorting shame can rob you of your identity. If you are a "mistake" or a "second-class citizen," other people's opinions are more important than your own. Their opinions of you become your sole measure of who you are.

Even success cannot overcome this shame, which tells you that you don't deserve success—or good things. You may fear others will find out about the "real you." Because of the shame, you might work to undermine any success that comes your way.

Shamed people tend to be angry in their powerlessness against other people—who matter more than they do.

A person's sense of distorting shame can have more than personal effects.

People who have grown up on shame often thrive on shaming others. Shamed people marry each other, and then they raise their children in an atmosphere of shame. The shame-shifting curse can follow to the third and fourth generations.

What can cover or fill our shame? Addictions, mood-altering experiences, which by definition are "out of control." We look for a temporary balm to soothe our shame—or loneliness and abandonment. But that awful hurt won't go away; the hole inside won't be filled, so we keep going back for more balm. It may be an emotional relationship; it may be sexual addiction; it may be alcohol or drugs; it may be *food*.

When you are in shame, you will "secretize" your needs. If you are eating-dependent, at some point—long before you had any choice about it—you began to meet a legitimate emotional need in an illegitimate way—with food.

135

Compulsive overeating is one coping skill that can numb the pain. Obsessive dieting may be a means of trying to take control. As we grow, as our lives become more complicated and stressful, the stress-reducing "demand" for food increases.

Most adult children with eating dependencies started out overeating as a response to stress. Their dependency on food formed as a way of protecting themselves from a pain that, as children, they had no power to remove. As adults they continue overeating as a means of denying feelings and blocking the intimacy of close relationships.

Bridgette, Merritt and Dana all turned to food to meet the needs not met by their families.

Food was both an enemy and friend to Bridgette, something that evaded her control and yet something that served as a pressure valve for the stress of living a life of perfection. Food became an object of love and trust to Merritt. Dana simply found that overeating could be used as a sedative, to help numb the pain she felt, to help fill the vacuum in her lonely life.

For Bridgette, every binge started in the same way: She would feel like, but resist, eating something sweet. The feeling would continue to gnaw at her. With guilt fluttering in her conscience, she would run an errand and come home with cookies, frozen yogurt and cheesecake. She would tell herself, just one cookie, maybe two. Definitely not more than four. After she had eaten the entire bag of cookies, a piece of cheesecake and two big bowls of frozen yogurt, she would sit as if stunned and ask, "Why did I do that?" She would be full, uncomfortably full, with her stomach hurting and bloated. No matter what the time of night, Bridgette would force herself to ride the stationary bike to exhaustion to "work it off," resolving not to do it again.

Merritt turned to food because she had no way to gain attention or to get her needs met in her family. She had to find a way to feel better all by herself, a way to stay afloat in the midst of the storms at home. Basically, overeating had become Merritt's life preserver, everything her family wasn't. Food was readily available to her and something she could get for herself. It never let her down; she could always count on feeling better. Dieting to Merritt meant letting go of her life preserver. She feared she was drowning.

For Dana, overeating was an energy that could be expended to help numb the pain in her life. When emotion would start to rise up, be it rejection or anger or fear, food was a way to push it back down. Even the yo-yo dieting she began as a teenager was effective at sedating emotions; while dieting she could keep everything in her head and not deal with the hurt in her heart. As long as she was on The Diet, she could be thinking obsessively about what she couldn't eat or when she could eat next. This kept her from feeling. But once off the diet, Dana returned to food and overeating to fill the void.

Releasing the Past:
A Process, *Not* an Event!

Coming to terms with your family, your feelings and your past permits a freedom not only from the food trap but from the whole destructive system of behavior associated with it. When you get to the point where you can make an adult commitment to live your own life, to release the past, your relationship with food will take on a whole new character. And that's what we'll discuss in chapter 10.

A Different Kind of Family Tree

Some people find it helpful to sit down and analyze the relationships in their childhood family. Look at it as a new kind of family tree, linking relationships. This tool may enlighten you to the tapes that continue to play within you and the systems in which you may be caught. Consider these questions carefully:

1. Look at the relationships in your family, between your mother and dad, grandmother and grandfather, parent and children, sibling and sibling. What dynamics characterized each relationship?

2. Look at significant life events or family landmarks. What light did each shed on the dynamics of relationships?

3. What strengths did you learn from the family systems? From your mother? From your father?

4. What weaknesses or negative character traits did you learn?

5. What were the beliefs and motives of the family system?

6. What did your family teach you about God?

7. Describe your relationship with your parents now (even if they are no longer living).

What systems are making you powerless to break free of the food trap? Allow any new information that surfaces in this family tree to be transformed by the renewing of your mind.

TEN

WALKING FREE

Have you ever dropped a glass, shattering it into little pieces? Our lives are very much like those broken fragments.

Now, in your mind, picture a beautiful stained glass window. A marvelous work of art—made of pieces of broken glass, yet new and complete. With God's healing and restoration, you can walk in a new reality, made from the shattered pieces of your life.

The conditions in which we were raised often keep us from placing our trust in God or other people. But God promises His children rest, an opportunity to start over and to get in touch with the wounded child within.

Jesus said we must become as little children to enter the kingdom of God. With this in mind, we can look forward to having the hurting child within being touched with the power of the living God!

Who Are You?

Knowing who you are is critical for emotional well-being. You are not a mistake; you were created by the God of the universe. Each of us is an individual, highly unique and important to God. He created us perfectly and specifically according to His image. "Let us make man in our image, in our likeness, and let them rule" (Gen. 1:26). God's image is our basis for being. No matter what has been done to us, no matter what was stolen from us, we were created in the image of God. We do not *have* God's image; we *are* God's image.

How we see ourselves is all-important. It determines how we live, what we accomplish and how others treat us. When we don't feel valuable, it is not important to preserve our bodies. It is easy to be entrapped by abusive, destructive patterns.

If you consider yourself to be a mistake, how can you ever be repaired? If you believe yourself to be defective as a human being, all you can do is try to cover up the defect. As you believe you are worth healing, you are able to accept healing.

Read this verse from the Word of God prayerfully: "Before I formed you in the womb I knew you, before you were born I set you apart" (Jer. 1:5). God loved you enough to choose to adopt you. Knowing all about you, who you are, what you feel, what you've done, what's been done to you, He chose to adopt you as His beloved child.

Galatians 4:6 tells us, "God sent the Spirit of his Son into our hearts, the Spirit who calls out, 'Abba, Father.' " He sent His Son to restore us to the same type of Abba-Father relationship that Adam and Eve enjoyed before the fall. They had true fellowship; they enjoyed intimacy; they communicated with each other (they heard His voice). God *chose* to have this relationship with us.

You need only to receive the spirit of adoption from the heavenly Father, God. Know that He loves you. He receives and accepts us as we are with all our strengths and weaknesses.

Truths of Freedom

Though you *are not* responsible for what was done to you as a child, you *are* responsible for taking positive steps to do something about it right now! You are responsible for breaking the cycle.

You are not to blame for the wrong choices of other people. You were a child and you were a victim. But however much your experiences may affect your life—they don't have to *ruin* it.

Each day we must decide whom to believe. The enemy of life will cast a vote of hopelessness. The voice will say, "You can never change. Look at the life you've had, what you've done, what's been done to you." The enemy has come to steal and destroy. He tries to steal our hope and our self-worth to make us useless to God and to others.

But God also casts a vote! He will speak the truth into your life. His voice says that you have been created to be a mighty overcomer, that you are loved, that you need only receive His gift and trust Him.

Each of us has the deciding vote. You and I break the tie; with whom will we side? Let us cast our vote with God!

Accept your responsibility and begin to receive from Him. Just as you chose to believe the lie about yourself—that you are not who God says you are—you can now *choose* to receive God's healing and freeing power.

Take a Risk

As you grasp hold of God's love for you, I ask you to take another great leap of faith: Acknowledge your emotional dependency on food to at least one other human being.

The way out of shame is to meet it face to face, to embrace it, to bring it out in the open. It's easy to miss deep inner healing, because we lack the courage to be vulnerable with another person. But trust is vital to healing. As long as we deny a problem exists, we can continue in it. Shame has a way of wrapping us in a secret, hidden cocoon. If our secrets are revealed, we're sure we will be rejected—and shamed further.

But God wants to meet our needs through relationships: a vital, personal relationship with Him and an honest relationship with at least one other human.

God created us with a natural need for acceptance and to be understood. That need is fulfilled through His complete and unconditional acceptance of us through His Son. Remember, we are adopted children! There is no greater form of unconditional love than to be chosen as His very own. He has continued to fulfill that acceptance by building a family of believers, a household of faith, that will love your Father with you and love you as well.

The apostle Paul admonished Christians to "carry each other's burdens" (Gal. 6:2). In another epistle where he is speaking of the unity of the church, he says to speak "the truth in love" so that we might "in all things grow up into him who is the Head, that is, Christ. From him the whole body, joined and held together by every supporting ligament, grows and builds itself up in love, as each part does its work" (Eph. 4:15-16).

The Holy Spirit often uses other discerning people to help us see our underlying problems. You'll want to choose your confidante prayerfully. It may be one or more trusted friends. It may be a counselor at your church. It may be a professional therapist. I encourage my patients who are dealing with issues such as incest, sexual abuse and alcohol in the family to seek professional counseling and therapy. These are deeply painful issues that affect every part of the being. A professional counselor has the skills to guide your walk through painful memories.

Not everyone needs a professional counselor—but a person with whom you can share your secret is vitally important. When you are ready to come out of hiding and go for help, you are saying, "I am worth helping."

I have mentioned the success of Alcoholics Anonymous, and many other twelve-step groups address other addictive diseases. These are not merely self-help groups that enable people to stop compulsive behavior. They teach people how to receive healing and live productively, as the twelve steps foster relationships of unconditional love and acceptance.

Nonjudgmental relationships—whether they are with trusted friends, a counseling support group, a small home-care group or a ministry team—show wounded people that they can trust again. They reflect God's love for us. Fellowship with a God-given new family can meet needs for intimacy and build up our self-esteem in ways that a family of origin may never be able to.

While human support is vital to breaking free from the food trap, know that, while others can *care*, they cannot *fix*. As food is not our ultimate comforter, neither are people our ultimate source of health and well-being. People will never be able to anticipate your needs quite as fast as you'd like. No one is at your side twenty-four hours a day. Loved ones can be taken from us through death.

The psalmist David knew this when he said, "Though my

father and mother forsake me, the Lord will receive me" (Ps. 27:10). That's the same writer who penned the promise of comfort: "The Lord is my shepherd, I shall not be in want...He restores my soul" (Ps. 23:1,3). In Pauline terms that would be "He renews my mind"!

Facing Your Feelings

Facing or embracing your past and your shame involves allowing yourself to feel emotions that you bottle up—or stuff with food.

As we humans were created, we can't ignore our feelings. They don't just "go away" because we deny them. If repressed, feelings linger and grow stronger and become a driving force in a life.

Remember: Birds fly, fish swim and people feel!

All feelings are legitimate; there is nothing good or bad about any of them. They are *all* part of who we humans were created to be. Emotions produce energy. And if we don't release that energy, we must work to keep it in.

Feelings stuffed inside can come out "sideways" through physical ailments—headaches, joint and muscle pain, an inability to sleep. Instead of crying, we get headaches. Instead of saying we don't want to go someplace with someone, we get stomach cramps. Instead of saying no to another work project, we push ourselves to exhaustion and develop high blood pressure—or we overeat. Our bodies react whether we like it or not. The unreleased energy robs us of our well-being by causing increased tension, anxiety or depression. *If you don't express, then you must repress and become depressed. Depression is emotion that has been frozen.*

Picture the emotional you as a teacup in the center of your soul. Every unexpressed emotion gets poured into the teacup. Day after day you allow unexpressed and unidentified feelings to drip into the cup until it is filled to the brim. Then, at some bizarre moment, maybe when the coat hangers won't separate properly, the whole teacup spills out, emptying in a torrent of rage. You really aren't that angry about the coat hangers, but heaven help the coat hangers, your closet and any poor soul who happens to be in the house. Feelings that aren't expressed properly will ultimately be expressed improperly!

To prevent emotions from building up internal barriers, allow yourself to feel whatever feelings are inside of you; don't judge the energy as good or bad. The feelings are simply a readout on where you are in life.

Rather than keeping feelings in, we can identify them and then *choose* to express them in an active, positive way. Our feelings do not have to control us; they must not dictate or control behaviors. Just because we are angry doesn't mean we have to scream and hurt someone. Just because we feel rejected doesn't mean we have to withdraw. We can release the energy in a number of positive ways: writing, creating something with our hands, singing, talking—exercising! Permit yourself to feel the energy and process it.

Journaling emotions (rather than stuffing them). Keeping a journal can be a positive way to express your feelings. In the privacy of these pages you can frankly say what you are feeling.

That's not for me, you may protest. Maybe you don't have the time—or the privacy. What if the journal fell out of the car and was picked up by a stranger? Worse yet, what if your children or spouse got ahold of it?

Look again. Are your protests really excuses? Finding ten extra minutes in a day is a matter of rearranging priorities. What if you left the lunchroom early or went to bed late? You can buy diary books with keys and locks. If you must guard the key, put it in a pillow case at the bottom of a pile in the linen closet. There are ways to dissolve excuses that rob you of the enormous release that comes in keeping a journal. Slowly your self-consciousness will fade, and you will be able to write out more and more of the feelings and thoughts that flood your inner soul and spirit.

Later, as you reread your journal entries, you will discover a you that you never knew. You can come to know an enormous part of your inner being and grasp hold of a freedom that comes with honesty. What a revelation it can be!

How to Journal

I use an inexpensive spiral-bound notebook found at an office supply store or where school supplies are sold. One of these provides enough space for two to three months of journaling. Of course any empty book will do, even one you make in a three-ring binder.

I write almost every day. Because I look at journaling as a gift of time to myself, I almost feel cheated when I miss a day for some reason.

What do I write about? I often start with *what* has happened to me, but I don't stop there. I write about how I feel about what has happened—or what might happen in the future.

You can write about your fears, inadequacies, regrets, joys, hopes and discoveries. When you feel happy, write it down. When you feel sad or angry or rejected, tell your "Dear Diary."

Let your journal help you identify what you're feeling. The act of writing has a way of forcing you to pinpoint—name— vague, free-floating anxiety or pain. Believe me, there is an enormous power that comes in names. Once you name how you feel about something, you begin to take power over it. It is no longer an unknown attacker.

By identifying and naming your feelings, you are giving yourself a chance to choose how best to process them. Remember, feeling an emotion is not sinful. It is what we do with the feeling that takes us toward or away from God's wholeness. As you write about a feeling—of anger or hurt or resentment—you can start to let go of it. As you process it, you gain a new perspective about the situation that caused the feeling in the first place. Why did a certain encounter trigger such a feeling? Did it remind you of something in your childhood? Some former pain? Did it make you feel shamed or inadequate? If so, why? Did you want to eat to cover or smooth the pain of the encounter?

What, if anything, should you do about the cause of the feeling, about the effects of any accompanying negative thoughts or behaviors? Is there a problem you need to solve? Did you misunderstand someone? Is it necessary or appropriate to discuss a point of tension with another person? How? When?

These and similar questions can be answered only in a still, quiet time. Your journal can be a tool to help you hear God's call to wholeness and freedom

It may be enough to feel the emotion and acknowledge it. Whatever the case, don't cling to unhealthy feelings. Letting go of them provides you with the space and energy for God-given joy, happiness and freedom.

Spiritual and emotional wellness is not the absence of problems. Far from it! Spiritual and emotional wellness is the ability to handle problems in a healthy way.

Choose Forgiveness

As you write out your feelings, submit each one to the healing, forgiving Holy Spirit.

You can never go back and relive your early life, but God

147

can restore what has been eaten away. The two major problems that result in emotional captivity are 1) the failure to receive forgiveness and 2) the failure to give forgiveness. Stacks of unforgiveness, like bricks, add up and weight us down.

There is a godly way to deal with all these hurts from the past. It is through *godly sorrow*, grieving for the loss of God's glory. Second Corinthians 7:10 says, "Godly sorrow brings repentance that leads to salvation and leaves no regret, but worldly sorrow brings death." Godly sorrow allows God's grace to be worked within us.

God wants to reach down into that child's heart of yours and lift your burden. Open your wound and pour out what you feel to God. Be totally honest and share every hurt with Him. Tell Him how you feel. He wants to heal you and comfort you.

In the Beatitudes Jesus said, "Blessed are those who mourn" (Matt. 5:4). By getting in touch with your pain over what was and what was not in your past and releasing that pain through proper grieving, you can gain a sense of closure to that part of your life. Know that the things that happened to you broke the heart of God; God cried over what was done to you. Grieve for that. Say good-bye to your childhood and grieve for that loss. Those who grieve well, live well, as they walk into abundant life.

I've seen that many people find it helpful to write a private letter to their primary caretaker while growing up. This is a letter they will never mail, and it tells their version of the hurts received as a child. They identify emotional or physical needs that were not met.

Such a letter can help you grieve for what you wanted and needed but didn't receive.

One client shared her letter with me and gave me permission to share it with you.

Dear Mommy and Daddy,

My counselor asked me to write you and tell you what I wanted and needed most from you, but you could never give me.

Daddy, I needed you to be there for me. I don't mean just at home; you were there, in body, every night. But I don't ever remember you even talking to me, or hugging me, or really even noticing me unless I had done something bad that day. You were always so mad and tired. I needed you to look at me. I needed to know that I was lovable. I needed to know that *you* loved me.

Mommy, you were always so faithful to provide me with everything I needed: You washed and ironed my clothes; the house was always spotless; you cooked wonderful food for us. But I needed you to listen to me. I needed you to care about how I felt, not just what I should do. I needed you to say you loved me. I needed you to show you loved me.

I know that all of these needs are still there because it hurts so much to write this letter to you.

But I am asking the Lord to heal these hurts. I can never be your little girl again to get these needs met.

I need to grow up now.

I love you,

Your daughter

Once the transgressions are on paper, ask the Lord to work in your spirit, loosing any unforgiveness you harbor. Grieving and forgiving often go hand in hand. You'll find that godly sorrow goes far beyond forgiving and surrendering resentment; it allows healing for open wounds. Walk in His mercy. Release the people who were the vehicles of your shame; release them to God, who wraps His loving purposes around our hurts to change them.

I love the Old Testament story of Joseph. Now there was a man who had reason to resent, even hate, his brothers who had sold him off as a slave. Years later, when Joseph met them again face to face, he was graced to see God's redeeming perspective on the situation. Speaking to his brothers Joseph said, "You intended to harm me, but God intended it for good to accomplish what is now being done" (Gen. 50:20). Joseph did not hold onto any bitterness against his family, nor did he blame God for painful experiences, which included years in prison because of a woman's false accusations.

Sometimes it is easier to blame an unseen God for our hurts and abandonments than to blame the people we grew up with. We transfer anger and mistrust toward our parents onto God: "God, why did You let this happen to me? If You were a loving, almighty God, You could have prevented this." Because God did not allow us a perfect childhood, we judge Him as weak. We believe the lie:

1) God cannot or will not meet our needs.

2) If we get our needs met in an unhealthy or sinful way, we will not experience any negative consequences.

3) We need to be our own god. If we're going to get our needs met, we better meet them ourselves, with our own systems for coping.

But the truth is that God is in the redemption business. Psalm 103:2-5 holds this promise: "Praise the Lord, O my soul, and forget not all his benefits. He forgives all my sins and heals all my diseases; he redeems my life from the pit and crowns me with love and compassion. He satisfies my desires with good things, so that my youth is renewed like the eagle's.'' He does this as we release our inadequacies—our very lives—to Him.

If shame keeps cropping up, verbally pass that shame back to the enemy of life, the father of lies. *It is his.* He is the one who shames and accuses.

Second Corinthians 4:1-2 says, ''Therefore, since through God's mercy we have this ministry, we do not lose heart. Rather, we have renounced secret and shameful ways; we do not use deception, nor do we distort the word of God.'' When the enemy tries to deliver shame and bitterness to your door, refuse to sign for it. He can knock all day, but you can refuse the package! Stir up the gift of God and remember God's perspective.

Katie began to break free of the food trap when she started identifying the unhealthy emotional and spiritual seeds that had been sown into her life.

Her family life had planted seeds of low self-worth that determined how she lived her life. Because she never attached value to her thoughts and feelings, she had no reason to treat her body in any way other than as an object to be scorned. As a child Katie learned to love food because it made her feel better. As a teen she learned to hate it because it made her fat. But as Katie realized that eating didn't make everyone fat, she concluded she must be as defective as she always had felt. Her relationship with God reflected her relationship with her parents. She felt she could get God to love her only if she didn't make trouble and did good things. She didn't love herself, so why should God love her?

As Katie named the unmet needs of her childhood and grieved for them, her emotional vacuum began to fill up with the love of God for her. She stopped blaming God for making her the way He did. She began to accept the fact that she was made perfect in His image. She embraced God's perspective of herself, as a valued treasure, a precious child.

Walking in freedom for Katie meant eating in a way that met her needs physically—so that she could let her newly restored relationships with God, herself and others meet her spiritual and emotional needs. Food could no longer be the protective barrier between Katie and the world, between Katie and God.

Take Time for Renewal

God wants to renew our minds, show us His perspective; but He works progressively over time, and He provides healing as we give Him time. Even Jesus required private time to maintain His peace: "The news about him spread all the more, so that crowds of people came to hear him and to be healed of their sicknesses. But Jesus often withdrew to lonely places and prayed" (Luke 5:15-16).

To succeed in our walk in freedom, we must continually affirm God's vote for our success. I have found three ways in my life to do this:

I take time to divert daily. This is a special time for me to pray, a special time for me to listen. My life is so full of demands that I must have regular, replenishing investments from God. It requires quiet to hear the gentle voice of God in my spirit. Diverting from everything for even twenty to thirty minutes gives me this quiet time.

I take time to withdraw weekly. I need a special time to be refreshed with the weekly Sabbath rest. I am on the go so much that sometimes I feel like a human "doing." All this doing is a trap for me, because it keeps me too busy to deal with the issues of the heart—too busy to notice and too busy to feel. I can easily slip into my "Scarlett O'Hara" mode (tucking needs away till a tomorrow that never comes).

My Sabbath rest gives me the chance to return to what I was created to be: a human *being*. It is a chance to review my activities and goals and evaluate them according to the purposes God has placed in my heart.

I joyfully take time annually to abandon my regular schedule. I need, and long for, a special time away, a "re-creation" time for God to speak anew into my life. When I am in God's created world, walking on a beach, hiking in the mountains or just gazing into His star-studded sky, I sense anew that I am a part of something much larger than me or my challenges in life. It brings unexpected peace and repair of the woundings of life.

A Daily Decision

I often think of one story about Winnie the Pooh and Piglet. One day the two were walking through the forest, and Piglet asked Pooh a question. "Pooh, what is the first thing you think of when you get up in the morning?"

Pooh answered, "I wonder what I will have for breakfast. Why? What is the first thing you think of when you wake up?"

Piglet answered, "I dream about what exciting thing will happen to me today!"

Do you face each day with a breakfast vision, or is each day an exciting adventure? As you believe God for vision and purpose, you will find fulfillment without getting sidetracked by the refrigerator.

As you embark on your journey to freedom and wellness, your decision—to commit yourself wholly to doing it God's way—must be renewed daily. Come to Him, seek His ways, ask His guidance, and He will guide, comfort, encourage and strengthen you.

There's a paradox to self-control. On one hand it is a matter of the will. We must *choose* to look to God for His power. And then we see that self-control is a fruit of His Spirit: "The fruit of the Spirit is love, joy, peace, patience, kindness, goodness, faithfulness, gentleness and self-control" (Gal. 5:22-23). You see, *self*-control comes only through *Spirit*-control. Control is something God does through us as we align our souls and bodies with His truth.

You might be tempted to turn back to food as the healing balm, but you know that it just doesn't work! God cannot comfort you unless you allow Him to. If you turn to food, you're not turning to Him. Trust Him to fulfill His promise.

Freedom comes in allowing God to meet your needs and desires in His way, in His timing.

Once you receive freedom, you can begin to give it away. We cannot give what we do not have. We cannot share love till we have love or share joy till we have joy or share freedom till we are free. As Jesus told His disciples: "Freely you have received, freely give" (Matt. 10:8).

My loving Father, reveal to me what it means to draw on Your power, to receive Your power, to walk in Your freedom—every day of the year.

PART IV:

PRACTICAL TIPS
FOR STAYING
ON TRACK

ELEVEN

THE PRACTICAL SIDE OF CHANGING BEHAVIOR

This chapter is designed to give you tips for living *well* in a world that doesn't. Here are tips to stay free over food in a world that revolves around it. Here are guidelines to help you entertain and be entertained—to enjoy food without being captive to it. You *can* eat out healthfully without having to take your own food with you.

Changes toward a life-style of wellness include your attitudes and relationship with food. To live free over food *and* dieting does not require you to carry around a calorie counter or scales and measuring cups. It requires a mind-set that enables you to make good food choices, regardless of your situation. It means being able to enjoy food without abusing it It means not walking around feeling deprived!

For the Cook of the House

Breaking the tasting chain. A lot of a cook's eating is not done consciously. While cooking or cleaning off the table, it's easy to pop in a taste of this, a bite of that, a little more of this and a spoonful of that. But all those "tastes" can add up to an entire meal's worth of calories! While cleaning the table, we fight our childhood teachings about wasting food. (You need to clean your plate to help save the starving children in Asia.)

Here are several tips to help you break the tasting chain:

- If you feel you must taste the dish you are preparing so you can adjust the spices, keep a measuring teaspoon available for the purpose. This will limit the amount you test. Keep track of the exact measure of what spices you add to a recipe. Once you get a recipe "just right," record exactly how much you used. Next time you will be able to trust the recipe without "having" to taste-test it.

- Cleaning up from a meal can cause as much harm as cooking it. Mom wasn't exactly giving you the facts when she said that cleaning your plate would save the lives of starving children. Your unhealthiness from overeating has never helped the hunger effort. If you want to aid these children, send money or support a charity. Do not overeat!

    Think of it this way: Wasting food is wasting food, whether it be in a body that doesn't need it or in a trash can. The difference: It doesn't hurt the trash can, but it does hurt your health.

- To make matters easier, serve up food at the stove, not family-style, which leads to the clean-out-the-bowl habit and makes portion control difficult, if not impossible. Seal leftovers and put them away before you sit down to eat. This way "going for more" requires more effort. *Even practice leaving a few bites on your plate*, to put a dent in the clean-plate syndrome.

Time-saving tips. Few people these days have the time or inclination to spend every afternoon preparing the dinner meal. Actually, lack of time can be a major obstacle to a wellness strategy. If your philosophy is "If it takes longer to cook it than to eat it, forget it!" then these tips are for you.

- When you cook, do so in abundance, then freeze properly portioned leftovers in freezer bags, providing quick meals when you need them.
- Keep two empty shoeboxes in your freezer and use them to store your ready-made meals. Put main-dish portions in one box, complements to the meal (rice, pastas, vegetables) in the other box.
- Spend one hour each week preparing some of the basics that will make each night's meal a healthy delight with a minimum of effort.

  For example, cook a big pot of brown rice, which can be reheated as needed. Make a batch of tomato sauce for use with pasta or as a topping for meat or "pita pizzas." Cook a pot of beans for beans and rice.
- For extra-quick stir-fry, use frozen bags of assorted vegetable mixes. The vegetables are already precut and can be fully cooked in four minutes! Bags of frozen peas can also be used for a quick carbohydrate.
- For a basic, quick salad, tear romaine lettuce and top with a tomato, a no-oil Italian dressing and a sprinkle of Parmesan.
- Keep a bowl of raw vegetables marinating in no-oil Italian dressing for a quick salad. You can add a small can of tuna to make a main dish and cooked pasta to make a whole meal.

Tips for the Food Shopper

- Be sure to go shopping *after* you've eaten your healthy meal or snack; do not go to the grocery store with your blood sugars low and your appetite out of control.
- Make a list of what you plan to buy, and stick to that plan. If it's not on the list, it doesn't belong in your cart. Let grocery shopping be a time to look for foods that *benefit* your body.
- Don't buy health-robbing foods "for the family." If you don't eat them on the way home, you will probably hide them in the back of the cupboard and eat them later. From experience I can say that these foods never seem to get past the hands of the buyer.
- Resist the temptation to feed others the very foods you are choosing to avoid. Feeding your loved ones energy-robbing, health-robbing foods is not an appropriate expression of love. You are only contributing to their unhealthiness.

"Just Say No!"

"Just say no" has been a powerful campaign slogan warning children and teens against drug use. The irony of such a campaign is that we adults can't even say no to a chocolate chip cookie. How can we expect our children to say no to drugs? Peer pressure didn't die in high school. No matter what your age, you must learn—or remember—to say one simple word that tends to get stuck in the human throat: No.

I have my patients practice saying no to the rearview mirror while driving, to the bathroom mirror while shaving, even to their make-up mirrors. Just practicing the word, seeing the word form on their lips, prepares them to "just say no" to unhealthy choices.

When you're offered a food that doesn't fit into your wellness plan, there's no need to give reasons for your action; neither is there a need to feel guilty, especially when the offering person is someone who knows what efforts you are making to be free over food. A caring friend will respect your desire for freedom and will understand a simple "No, thank you."

Of course not every host (or family cook) is a supportive voice. You will hear discouraging and tempting comments: "Come on, you can splurge tonight. You deserve a little fun once in a while!" "Oh, just a little bit won't hurt." Even, "I think you're carrying this too far. You're in bondage to this nutrition thing."

Again, try to prepare yourself for people's negative response to the change in your life. Realize that feeding someone rich and "special" foods is one common way of expressing love to that person. As you show that you do not equate food with love, such cooks are likely to learn to express their love to you in alternate ways. Answer with a simple "No, thank you." It is your life and your choice for a life of freedom. Self-control is not bondage.

Never say, "I *can't* eat this"; instead say, "I don't care for any, thank you." Those words communicate strength and decisiveness *and* make a positive confession. The truth is, you *can* eat anything; there are just some foods that you choose not to.

Party Tips for Moderation

- Always eat a healthy snack before going to parties, open houses, and the like, so you can maintain control over your "appetite for the appetizers." You can more judiciously taste what you choose when you don't arrive famished.

- Never starve yourself on the day of a big party or meal. You will only throw off your metabolism and set yourself up for disaster. Instead maintain your small, evenly spaced meals throughout the day, which will keep your metabolism and appetite in better control.

- Never tell people you are dieting; it is self-sabotage. You will quickly be talked into eating everything. If you feel you must say anything, just say, "No, thank you." Don't look pitiful in a corner. (No one ever notices that the life of the party isn't eating.)

- Remember the problem is not the "big parties" but your day-by-day eating. Avoid the I've-blown-it-now syndrome.

Overcoming Setbacks: Avoiding the I've-Blown-It-Now Syndrome

Making changes in eating behavior is a lot like running a marathon; it takes pacing, consistency and endurance. Those who jump out ahead, trying to take a short cut, will either burn out or be disqualified. On the other hand, a runner can stumble again and again and still cross the finish line if he or she is determined to keep going. That runner just needs to keep his or her eyes more closely focused on the road out ahead and continue to put one foot in front of the other.

Be assured that one lapse in your new eating patterns does not ruin all the health you have gained through those patterns. Your health will never be ruined by one extravagant meal, one hot dog at a ball game or one slice of birthday cake; only fad diets can be "blown."

A lapse in your healthy life-style is just that—*a lapse*. It was one less-than-ideal choice that you made. Do not let it become a relapse, another relapse, another relapse—and finally a collapse, which is the I've-blown-it-now syndrome in a nutshell.

The sooner you realize that there's no atonement for a poorly chosen meal, the better off you'll be. Don't try to fast the next day, to punish yourself with restrictive dieting or take a laxative. Just choose to get back on track with your nutritious, healthy eating.

You can do this by listening to your body and how bad it feels after you've eaten foods that are not good for you. Your body has been designed so wonderfully that it will reinforce your choice to eat in a healthier style. The reason you are avoiding high-fat and highly sweetened foods is because they are wellness-robbers; no food is worth the GI distress, bloating and sluggishness you can expect.

If you are a scale-watcher, beware! The scale may reflect as much as three to four pounds of fluid retention following a lapse in your good eating. It is only temporary; your weight will stabilize after three or four days. Your feeling heavy and bloated should underscore the reasons why you are choosing to eat in a healthier way.

Know that you will walk through difficult, vulnerable times—the daily cares of this life, fatigue, personal obligations—that seem to draw you back to old, predictable patterns. Overcoming each difficult time will make the next time easier.

You will be living one day at a time and one meal at a time. Some days will work out as you desire, and some won't. The joys and rewards come from continuing to see changes in your attitudes, your body and your life!

TWELVE

EATING FREE

Living free of the food trap involves choosing a way of eating and living for a lifetime—*never a diet!* Even if you want to lose weight, the way you eat must be so comfortable that you can stay with it for the rest of your life.

Eating-behavior changes have no legals and cheatings, goods or bads, on its or off its. You only need to focus on eating healthy foods at the right time.

I have included the Have It Your Way meal plan from my book *Alive and Well in the Fast Food Lane* (coauthored with Carolyn Coats). It is designed to work with your body, providing you with a lifetime of high energy and wellness.

I am also giving you *Alive and Well*'s grocery list, to help you shop wisely, and recipes for perfect breakfasts, wonderful lunches and delicious and healthy dinners.

Remember, this is about freedom, not about dieting!

HAVE IT YOUR WAY
WEIGHT-LOSS MEAL PLAN FOR WOMEN

BREAKFAST   within 1/2 hour of arising

Complex Carbo:	1 slice of 100% whole wheat bread OR 1/2 whole wheat English muffin OR 3/4 cup cereal WITH raw bran added (Begin with 1 tsp. bran, gradually increasing to 2 Tbsp.)
Protein:	1 oz. low-fat cheese OR 1/2 cup plain non-fat yogurt OR 3/4 cup low-fat milk for cereal OR 1 egg (limit eggs to 3 times per week)
Simple Carbo:	1 small piece of fresh fruit

A.M. SNACK

Carbo:	3 whole grain crackers OR 1 piece of fruit OR 1 rice cake/Wasa
Protein:	1 oz. cheese/lean meat OR 1/2 cup non-fat yogurt (mix with 1 tsp. all-fruit jam)

LUNCH

Complex Carbo:	2 slices of bread OR 1 baked potato OR 10 crackers OR 1 whole wheat pita
Protein:	2 oz. low-fat cheese OR cooked poultry, fish, lean roast beef OR 1/2 cup cooked legumes
Simple Carbo:	1 small piece of fresh fruit OR 1 cup non-creamed soup
Free Munchie:	Raw vegetable salad, if desired, with no-oil dressing
Added Fat:	1 tsp. mayonnaise/margarine/olive or canola oil OR 1 Tbsp. salad dressing

AFTERNOON SNACK   Repeat earlier snack choices OR 1/4 cup trail mix

DINNER

Complex Carbo: 1/2 cup rice/pasta OR 1/2 cup starchy vegetable

Protein: 2 oz. cooked chicken, turkey, fish, seafood, lean roast beef OR 1/2 cup cooked legumes

Simple Carbo: 1 cup non-starchy vegetable OR 1 piece of fresh fruit

Free Munchie: Raw vegetable salad, if desired, with no-oil dressing

Added Fat: May use 1 tsp. margarine/olive oil OR 1 Tbsp. salad dressing

NIGHT SNACK   1 piece of fruit OR 3 cups microwave light popcorn

FREEBIES   Raw vegetables, mustard, vinegar, lemon juice

WEIGHT-MAINTENANCE MEAL PLAN FOR WOMEN AND WEIGHT-LOSS MEAL PLAN FOR MEN

BREAKFAST within 1/2 hour of arising

Complex Carbo: 2 slices of 100% whole wheat bread OR 1 whole wheat English muffin OR 1-1/2 cups cereal WITH raw bran added (begin with 1 tsp. bran, gradually increasing to 2 Tbsp.)

Protein: 2 oz. low-fat cheese OR 2 Tbsp. natural peanut butter OR 8 oz. low-fat milk for cereal OR 2 eggs—(limit eggs to two times a week)

Simple Carbo: 1 small piece of fresh fruit

A.M. SNACK

Carbo: 5 whole grain crackers OR 1 piece of fruit OR 2 rice cakes/Wasa

Protein: 2 oz. cheese/lean meat OR 2 Tbsp. natural peanut butter (limit peanut butter to once a day) OR 8 oz. plain, nonfat yogurt

LUNCH

Complex Carbo: 2 slices of bread OR 1 baked potato OR 1 whole wheat pita

Protein: 2-3 oz. low-fat cheese OR cooked poultry, fish, lean roast beef OR 3/4 cup cooked legumes

Simple Carbo: 1 small piece of fresh fruit OR 1 cup non-creamed soup

Free Munchie: Raw vegetable salad, if desired, with no-oil dressing

Added Fat: 1 tsp. mayonnaise/margarine/olive or canola oil OR 1 Tbsp. salad dressing

AFTERNOON SNACK

Repeat earlier snack choices OR 1/2 cup trail mix

DINNER

Complex Carbo: 1 cup rice/pasta OR 1 cup starchy vegetable

Protein:	3-4 oz. cooked chicken, turkey, fish, seafood, lean roast beef OR 1 cup cooked legumes
Simple Carbo:	1 cup non-starchy vegetable OR 1 piece of fresh fruit
Free Munchie:	Raw vegetable salad, if desired, with no-oil dressing.
Added Fat:	May use 1 tsp. margarine/olive oil OR 2 Tbsp. sour cream OR 1 Tbsp. salad dressing

NIGHT SNACK	1/2 cup cereal with 1/2 cup milk OR use any earlier snack

FREEBIES	Raw vegetables, mustard, vinegar, lemon juice, no-oil dressing

---

WEIGHT-MAINTENANCE MEAL PLAN FOR MEN

BREAKFAST	within 1/2 hour of arising
Complex Carbo:	2 slices of 100% whole wheat bread OR 1 whole wheat English muffin OR 1-1/2 cups cereal WITH raw bran added (begin with 1 tsp., gradually increasing to 2 Tbsp.)
Protein:	2 oz. low-fat cheese OR 2 Tbsp. natural peanut butter OR 8 oz. low-fat milk for cereal OR 2 eggs (limit eggs to twice per week)
Simple Carbo:	1 piece of fresh fruit

A.M. SNACK

Carbo: 5 whole grain crackers OR 1 piece of fruit OR 2 rice cakes OR 1 slice of bread

Protein: 2 oz. cheese/lean meat OR 2 Tbsp. natural peanut butter (limit peanut butter to once a day) OR 8 oz. plain, nonfat yogurt

LUNCH

Complex Carbo: 2 slices of bread OR 1 baked potato OR 1 whole wheat pita

Protein: 3-4 oz. low-fat cheese OR cooked poultry, fish, lean roast beef OR 1 cup cooked legumes

Simple Carbo: 1 piece of fresh fruit AND 1 cup non-creamed soup

Free Munchie: Raw vegetable salad, if desired, with no-oil dressing

Added Fat: 1 tsp. mayonnaise/margarine/olive or canola oil OR 1 Tbsp. salad dressing

AFTERNOON SNACK

Repeat earlier snack choices OR 3/4 cup trail mix

DINNER

Complex Carbo: 1 cup rice/pasta OR 1 cup starchy vegetable

Protein: 4 oz. cooked chicken, turkey, fish, seafood, lean roast beef OR 1 cup cooked legumes

Simple Carbo: 1 cup non-starchy vegetable AND 1 piece of fresh fruit

Free Munchie: Raw vegetable salad, if desired, with no-oil dressing

Added Fat: May use 2 tsp. margarine or olive oil OR 2 Tbsp. sour cream OR 2 Tbsp. salad dressing

NIGHT
SNACK
Any Power Snack (see page 59) OR 1/2 cup cereal with 1/2 cup milk OR use any earlier snack

FREEBIES Raw vegetables, mustard, vinegar, lemon juice

GROCERY LIST

GRAINS

- 100% whole wheat bread—Do not buy very thin or diet slice; look for "whole" as the first word in the ingredient list.
- Whole wheat English muffins and pita bread
- Whole wheat pasta and whole wheat pastry flour—may need to get from natural food store
- Brown rice
- Whole grain crackers
    Rye Krisp: 3 = 1 slice bread
    rice cakes: 2 = 1 slice bread
    Wasa crackers: 2 = 1 slice bread
    Kavli-Norwegian flatbread: 4 thins = 1 slice bread
    Harvest Crisp: 5 = 1 slice bread
    Wheatsworth—not 100% whole wheat and higher salt but good for variety: 5 = 1 slice bread

- Cereals
    Kellogg's Nutrigrain—Wheat, Corn and Almond
      Raisin
    shredded wheat, Shredded Wheat-N-Bran
    Raisin Squares
    puffed rice, puffed wheat, oatmeal, Wheatena
    Grape-nuts (concentrated: 1/4 cup = 3/4 cup
      other cereals)
- Oat bran
    Quaker, Arrowhead Mills Oat Bran Cereal (from
      natural food store or grocery store)
- Wheat bran—Use raw, unprocessed available at natural
  food store or Quaker Raw Unprocessed Bran available
  at grocery store

DAIRY AND DELI

- Skim or 1 percent low-fat milk
- Plain nonfat OR low-fat yogurt
- Eggs
- Butter or 100 percent corn oil margarine (squeeze type
  is best)
- Cheeses: All of these are available at grocery store; look
  for any cheese marked "part-skimmed milk."
    part-skimmed milk mozzarella
    light cream cheese
    Weight Watcher's Natural Cheddar, Kraft Natural Lite
      Cheddar, Laughing Cow reduced-calorie wedges
      (box cheese that doesn't require refrigeration)
    Lorraine Swiss at deli—Have it sliced on #9; each
      slice = 1 oz. You may also have turkey or roast
      beef sliced on #9.

low-fat cottage cheese (less than 2 percent fat)
farmer's cheese
ricotta—part skimmed
string cheese

MISCELLANEOUS

- Assorted variety of seasonal fresh fruits and vegetables, such as bananas, apples, oranges, melon, strawberries; romaine lettuce, broccoli, carrots, tomatoes, squash, white and sweet potatoes. Also buy raisins and canned, unsweetened applesauce and crushed pineapple.

- Mayonnaise—may use a tsp. of traditional mayonnaise OR 1 Tbsp. Miracle Whip Lite OR Kraft Light and Lively

- Olive oil, canola oil

- Natural peanut butter—may buy fresh ground at deli or from health food store

- Dry roasted, unsalted peanuts and shelled sunflower seeds for trail mix

- Low-calorie salad dressings—may prefer to use 1 Tbsp. regular dressing with lemon juice or vinegar
    Bernstein's Low-Calorie Cheese Italian or Vinaigrette; Kraft no-oil dressing; Barendorf's; and Pritikin's

- No-sugar jam—try Sorrell Ridge, Polaner Preserves or Smuckers' Simply Fruit (fruit only preserves)

PERFECT BREAKFASTS THAT ARE QUICK, EASY AND DELICIOUS!

Remember that breakfast is the "stick" that stokes your metabolic fire. You need more than just a piece of toast and coffee to give your day a "sunny beginning." Try the following breakfast ideas, a different one every day, for a wonderful variety of ways to start your day just right!

CHEESE DANISH

1/2 whole wheat English muffin
2 Tbsp. Philadelphia Lite Cream Cheese
2 Tbsp. raisins OR 1 Tbsp. Sorrell Ridge,
Polaner Preserves or Smuckers' Simply Fruit

Spread muffin with Lite cream cheese; if possible, warm in toaster oven. Top with raisins or preserves. (Another marvelous choice: mash 1/4 cup fresh berries and put on top of cheese and muffin.) Makes 1 serving.

1 complex CHO: muffin / 1 oz. protein: cheese
1 simple CHO: raisins

OATMEAL WITH A DIFFERENCE

1/3 cup old-fashioned oats	**1 Tbsp. raisins**
3/4 cup skim milk	**cinnamon**
1/4 cup unsweetened apple juice	**1/2 tsp. vanilla**

Bring milk, apple juice and oatmeal to a boil. Gently cook for 5 minutes, stirring occasionally. Add raisins, vanilla and cinnamon; let sit covered for 2-3 minutes to thicken. Makes 1 serving.

1 complex CHO: oats / 1 oz. protein: milk
1 simple CHO: juice and raisins

PEANUT BUTTER DANISH

1 slice 100 percent whole grain bread
2 Tbsp. natural peanut butter
1/2 banana

Slice banana lengthwise and place with inside facing down on the slice of bread. Top with peanut butter. Broil until peanut butter is slightly brown and bubbly. Surprise! Makes 1 serving.

1 complex CHO: bread / 1 oz. protein: peanut butter
1 simple CHO: banana

SUNDAY FRENCH TOAST

4 egg whites, lightly beaten
3/4 cup skim milk
1/4 cup unsweetened juice
1 tsp. vanilla
1/2 tsp. cinnamon
6 slices whole wheat bread
fruit preserves (no sugar) or mashed fresh fruit

Beat together egg whites, milk, juice, vanilla and cinnamon. Add bread slices one at a time, letting the bread absorb liquid in the process. May let sit for a few minutes. Spray non-stick skillet with cooking spray and heat. Gently lift the bread with spatula into skillet and cook until golden brown on each side. Serve topped with 1/2 cup fresh fruit or 1 Tbsp. preserves. Makes 6 servings. You can freeze the extras and pop them in the microwave on a busy morning.

1 complex CHO: bread / 1 oz. protein: eggs, milk
1 simple CHO: fruit

PERFECT BOWL OF CEREAL

3/4 cup approved cereal (see grocery list)
1/2 cup skim milk
1 Tbsp. unprocessed wheat bran AND 1 Tbsp. oat bran
1/2 cup fruit OR 1 small banana OR 2 Tbsp. raisins
  (1 tiny box)

1 complex CHO: cereal / 1 oz. protein: milk
1 simple CHO: fruit

BREAKFAST SHAKE

1/2 cup frozen fruit*   **2 Tbsp. nonfat dry milk**
1 cup skim milk   **2 Tbsp. wheat germ**
1 tsp. vanilla   **1 Tbsp. oat bran**

Blend frozen fruit in blender. Add remaining ingredients and continue blending till smooth.

1 complex CHO: wheat germ and bran / 1 oz. protein: milk
1 simple CHO: fruit

*Don't throw away your very ripe bananas. Freeze them in freezer bags and use for your shakes.

BREAKFAST PARFAIT

1/2 cup plain, nonfat yogurt
1/2 cup blueberries OR 1 small mashed banana OR
  1/2 cup unsweetened crushed pineapple (strawberries
  may be too tart)
1/4 cup Grape-nuts
cinnamon

Layer yogurt, fruit and cereal parfait-style into tall parfait glass. Sprinkle with cinnamon and ENJOY!

1 complex CHO: cereal / 1 oz. protein: yogurt
1 simple CHO: fruit

EATING FREE

CHEESE APPLE SURPRISE

1 slice whole wheat bread	**1/2 apple, thinly sliced**
1 Tbsp. raisins	**1 oz. mozzarella cheese**

Top bread with apple and raisins. Place cheese on apple-raisin layer. Broil until cheese is bubbly. Makes 1 serving.

1 complex CHO: bread / 1 oz. protein: cheese
1 simple CHO: apple and raisins

MUFFIN MAGIC

Oat bran muffin (your complex carbohydrate)
8 oz. skim milk or plain, nonfat yogurt (your protein)
Fresh fruit (your simple carbohydrate)

OAT BRAN MUFFINS

2-1/4 cups oat bran
1/4 cup honey
1-1/4 cups skim milk
2 egg whites
2 Tbsp. Puritan or safflower oil
1 Tbsp. baking powder
3/4 tsp. cinnamon
1/2 tsp. pumpkin or apple pie spice
1/4 tsp. salt
1/4 cup raisins

Preheat the oven to 425 degrees. Process the oat bran with large blade in food processor while mixing other ingredients (this will lighten up the muffins). Mix the milk, egg whites, honey and oil together. Add the baking powder, spices and salt to the bran in processor; blend. Add the liquid mixture and process just until blended. Add raisins.

Line muffin pans with paper baking cups, and fill with batter. Bake 15 to 17 minutes; test for doneness at 15 minutes

177

with a toothpick—it should come out moist but not wet. Makes 12 muffins. Store in a plastic bag to retain moisture. If you will not use these in three days, store in freezer and thaw one at a time.

Optional: Omit pie spice, 1/2 cup skim milk and raisins. Add 1 small can crushed pineapple and 1 small mashed banana.

WONDERFUL LUNCHES

Don't skip lunch, and don't get into a rut either! For a lunch that will refresh you and keep your energy high, try one of these delicious and fast complete meals.

SEAFOOD SALAD

1/2 cup water-packed tuna or salmon
1 tsp. of Dijon mustard
1 Tbsp. of reduced-calorie mayonnaise

1 stalk chopped celery
1/4 tsp. beau monde (optional)
1/4 tsp. dill
pepper to taste

Mix together ingredients. Serve on bed of torn romaine lettuce with 10 whole grain crackers and fresh fruit.

Complex CHO: crackers / protein: fish
Simple CHO: fruit / added fat: mayonnaise

PEANUT BUTTER AND BANANA SANDWICH

2 Tbsp. natural peanut butter (never, never commercial)
2 slices of whole wheat bread
1 small sliced banana

Complex CHO: bread / protein: peanut butter
Simple CHO: banana

CHEF'S SALAD

sliced veggies—as many as possible (try to have at least 5)
romaine lettuce
2 oz. chicken, turkey or Lorraine Swiss cheese

Toss vegetables with lettuce; top with meat or cheese. You may use croutons made by toasting 2 pieces whole wheat that have been sprinkled with garlic powder (not salt!). Cut these into cubes and store in jar or tin to have on hand. Serve with whole grain crackers and fresh fruit.

Complex CHO: crackers/croutons / protein: turkey
Simple CHO: fruit / added fat: 1 Tbsp. dressing

CHICKEN, TURKEY OR ROAST BEEF SANDWICH

2 oz. meat (trimmed of all fat)
2 slices whole wheat bread
1 tsp. mayonnaise and/or mustard
lettuce and sliced tomato

Spread bread with mayonnaise and/or mustard. Layer with meat of choice; top with lettuce and tomato. Serve with a delicious piece of fruit.

Complex CHO: bread / protein: turkey
Simple CHO: fruit / added fat: mayonnaise

CHICKEN OF THE LAND
OR SEA APPLE SANDWICH

1/2 cup water-packed tuna
   or chicken
1 small stalk of chopped celery
1 Tbsp. reduced-calorie mayonnaise
1 small chopped apple
1 whole wheat pita
romaine lettuce leaves

Mix together first 4 ingredients. Stuff into 2 halves of pita lined with lettuce.

Complex CHO: pita / protein: chicken
Simple CHO: fruit / added fat: mayonnaise

VEGGIE SANDWICH

1 whole wheat pita
2 oz. cheese (mozzarella, skimmed cheddar or Lorraine
   Swiss)
a few mushrooms and green pepper rings
sliced tomato

Stuff halved pita with 1 oz. cheese each and vegetables. Microwave on high for 2-3 minutes. Add a couple of tomato slices and be ready for a treat. Serve with a fruit juice spritzer (1/2 cup juice mixed with club soda or seltzer) over ice.

Complex CHO: pita / protein: cheese
Simple CHO: juice

HEALTHY HAMBURGER

1 whole wheat hamburger bun
3 oz. ground round or ground turkey patty
lettuce and tomato slices

Grill or broil hamburger patty (the fat will drain through rack and will cook meat down to 2 to 2-1/2 oz.) Place on whole wheat bun with lettuce, tomato slices, mustard and a small amount of ketchup (if desired). One pound of ground round = five 2 oz. patties after cooking. Serve with melon slices.

Complex CHO: bun / protein: hamburger
Simple CHO: melon

CARROT-CHEESE MELT

2 coarsely grated carrots   **2 slices whole wheat bread**
1/2 cup grated mozzarella   **1 tsp. mayonnaise**
cheese

Mix together carrots and cheese. Spread bread with 1 tsp. mayonnaise and top with carrot-cheese mix. Grill in nonstick skillet till cheese melts. Add tomato slices, lettuce (and even alfalfa sprouts!).

Complex CHO: bread / protein: cheese
Simple CHO: carrots / added fat: mayonnaise

EASY, DELICIOUS
AND HEALTHY DINNERS

Sometimes having a foundation from which to work can be invaluable! Here are eight meals you can use for starters. They are perfectly balanced; everyone will like them; and they are easy! Freeze properly portioned leftovers in freezer bags for quick meals when you need them most!

OVEN-BAKED CHICKEN—your protein
PEAS ROSEMARY—your complex carbohydrate and
  meal's added fat

181

STEAMED CABBAGE—your simple carbohydrate
CARROT-RAISIN SALAD—the rest of your simple
carbohydrate

OVEN-BAKED CHICKEN

1 egg, lightly beaten
1 cup Nutrigrain wheat cereal, crushed
1/4 tsp. pepper
6 chicken half-breasts, deboned and skinned
1 Tbsp. water
1/4 tsp. garlic powder
1/4 tsp. seasoned salt (optional)

Mix together egg and water in shallow dish; set aside. Combine crushed cereal and spices. Dip chicken in egg mixture, then dredge in cereal mixture, coating well. Arrange in baking pan coated with cooking spray. Bake, uncovered, at 350 degrees for 45 minutes, or until tender. Yields 6 servings each, giving you your protein and part of your complex carbohydrate.

PEAS ROSEMARY

1 pkg. frozen peas,   1/4 tsp. pepper
  cooked and drained   1 tsp. rosemary
2 tsp. corn oil margarine   1/4 tsp. salt (optional)
2 cloves minced garlic   1/4 cup chopped onion

Saute garlic and onion in margarine till tender. Add rosemary, salt and pepper and continue to saute one more minute. Toss with peas. Makes 4 servings; one serving would be your complex carbohydrate and your meal's added fat.

CARROT-RAISIN SALAD A LA DIFFERENCE

1 lb. coarsely grated carrots
1 cup firm plain low-fat
  yogurt
1/2 cup raisins

2 medium apples, grated
1/2 cup crushed
  unsweetened pineapple

Combine all ingredients and chill. Makes 4 servings; 1/2 cup serving counts as part of your simple carbohydrate.

MARVELOUS MEATLOAF—your protein and part of
  your complex carbohydrate
CORN ON THE COB—your complex carbohydrate
COLORFUL GREEN BEANS—your simple carbohydrate
ROMAINE SALAD—your healthy munchie

MARVELOUS MEATLOAF

2 lbs. ground round or ground turkey
2 cups old-fashioned oats
3/4 cup minced onion
1/4 green pepper, minced
2 eggs, slightly beaten
1/2 tsp. each salt and pepper
1 Tbsp. worchestershire sauce
1 tsp. dry mustard
1/4 cup skim milk
3/4 cup tomato sauce

In large bowl, mix together all ingredients except for 1/2 cup of the tomato sauce. Shape meat into 2 loaves and place in loaf pans sprayed with cooking spray. Spread the additional 1/2 cup tomato sauce on top. Bake in 400-degree oven for 40 minutes. Makes 12 servings; a 3 oz. serving counts as your protein.

COLORFUL GREEN BEANS

1 lb. green beans
1/2 cup chopped onion
1/2 tsp. salt (optional)
2 medium tomatoes, peeled
  and cut into 8 wedges

2 tsp. olive oil
1/2 cup chopped celery
1/4 tsp. pepper

Remove strings from beans; wash and cut diagonally into 2'' pieces. Heat oil in skillet, add onion and celery to skillet and saute until tender; add beans, salt and pepper. Cover and simmer 10 minutes, stirring occasionally. Add tomato; cover and cook an additional 5 minutes. Makes 4 servings; each serving counts as your simple carbohydrate and your meal's added fat.

HAWAIIAN CHICKEN—your protein
WILD RICE PILAF—your complex carbohydrate
GREEN BEANS AND MUSHROOMS—your simple
  carbohydrate
SLICED TOMATOES—your healthy munchie

HAWAIIAN CHICKEN

1/3 cup unsweetened
  pineapple juice
1/3 cup low sodium
  soy sauce
1/3 cup sherry (optional)

2 cloves garlic
1 Tbsp. parsley
ground pepper to taste
4 skinned chicken breasts

Mix all but chicken. Marinate chicken breasts (skinned, deboned and split lengthwise) for 3-4 hours or overnight. (The marinade adds no significant calories.) Grill. Makes 4 servings; one serving would be your protein.

WILD RICE PILAF

1 tsp. olive oil
1 medium onion, chopped
1 clove minced garlic
1 stalk celery, chopped
2-1/3 cups chicken broth

1/4 cup wild rice
3/4 cup brown rice
1/4 tsp. salt (optional)
1 Tbsp. parsley

Saute vegetables in medium saucepan with 1 tsp. olive oil. Add broth and optional salt; bring to boil and add rices. Boil for one minute—reduce heat and simmer for 45 minutes until the liquid is absorbed. Garnish with parsley. Makes six 1/2 cup servings; one serving would be your complex carbohydrate.

GREEN BEANS WITH MUSHROOMS

1 Tbsp. olive oil
1 clove minced garlic
1/2 lb. washed mushrooms
1/2 tsp. rosemary
1/2 tsp. basil

1 Tbsp. parsley
1/2 tsp. salt (optional)
1/4 tsp. pepper
1 lb. steamed green beans

Saute garlic and mushrooms in olive oil for 5 minutes. Add spices and simmer covered for another 3-4 minutes. Toss well with beans. Makes 6 servings; each counts as your simple carbohydrate and fat.

SALMON OF THE DAY—your protein
BAKED SWEET POTATO—your complex carbohydrate
STEAMED BROCCOLI—your simple carbohydrate
WALDORF SALAD—your simple carbohydrate

BAKED SALMON IN A POUCH

1/4 cup cider vinegar	4 salmon steaks, 1 inch thick
1/2 tsp. Dijon mustard	1 sliced green pepper
1/2 tsp. dillweed	1 thinly sliced tomato
1/4 tsp. minced garlic	1 minced scallion

Combine vinegar, mustard, dill and garlic in glass baking dish. Add salmon and marinate for 10 minutes. Turn salmon over and marinate 10 minutes more. Cut four 8" x 8" sheets of aluminum foil. For each serving, place a salmon steak in the center of foil. Distribute peppers, tomatoes, scallions and dill on top. Drizzle with marinade. Fold and pinch foil to seal fish inside. Bake at 375 degrees for 15 to 20 minutes. Remove from foil and serve immediately. Makes 4 servings; each gives you protein.

POACHED SALMON

1-1/2 cups white wine or chicken broth	1/2 cup water
1 lemon, sliced	1 onion, sliced
1 tsp. dried dillweed	4 sprigs parsley
1/4 tsp. pepper	extra sliced lemon

4 1-inch thick salmon steaks or other fish fillets

Combine all ingredients except fish and additional lemon slices in a large skillet. Bring to a boil; cover, reduce heat and simmer 10 minutes. Add salmon steaks or fillets; cover and simmer 8 minutes or until fish flakes easily. Remove from skillet; garnish with lemon slices. Makes 4 servings; each gives you protein.

GRILLED SALMON

1/2 tsp. allspice
1 tsp. cardamon (optional)
2 cloves garlic, minced
additional lime slices

1/3 cup lime juice
1-1/3 lbs. salmon steaks,
about 1 inch thick

Combine spices with garlic and lime juice. Arrange salmon in a single layer in shallow dish; cover with marinade. Let stand for 15 minutes, then turn over and let stand for 15 minutes more. Grill salmon for 5 minutes per side or until it flakes easily. Makes 4 servings; 1 serving counts as protein.

SALMON LOAF

1 medium onion, chopped
3/4 cup old-fashioned oats
  (uncooked)
1/2 cup unprocessed bran
15-1/2 oz. can salmon, drained
1 cup buttermilk
1/4 tsp. garlic powder

2 eggs, lightly beaten
1 Tbsp. parsley
1/2 tsp. dill
1/2 tsp. salt (optional)
1/4 tsp. pepper
lemon & parsley to
  garnish

Mix together all ingredients. Pack into an 8-1/2 x 4-1/2 inch bread pan sprayed with nonstick spray. Bake at 350 degrees for 40 minutes, until firm. Garnish with lemon wedges and parsley. Makes 6 servings; each serving counts as your protein and part of your complex carbohydrate.

WALDORF IN DISGUISE

2 large apples, in chunks
1/2 cup unsweetened
  pineapple chunks
1/2 stalk chopped celery
1/2 cup sliced carrots

1 sliced green pepper
1 small orange,
  sectioned
1/4 cup raisins

Combine with dressing and chill; top with 1/2 cup chopped nuts. Makes six 1/2 cup servings; one serving will count as your simple carbohydrate and with nuts, as your meal's added fat.

Dressing:

3/4 cup plain low-fat yogurt	**1/2 cup orange juice**
juice from 1/2 lemon	**dash salt and cinnamon**

Mix a lot of dressing at one time and keep in refrigerator for a wonderful fruit topping.

CHILI CON CARNE—your protein, complex and simple
  carbohydrates
ROMAINE SALAD—your healthy munchie
SLICED MELON—more simple carbohydrate

CHILI CON CARNE*

1 lb. ground round or	**1 tsp. basil**
ground turkey	**2-3 tsp. chili powder**
1 tsp. olive oil	**1 tsp. salt (optional)**
1 cup chopped onion	**1/8 tsp. pepper**
2 cloves crushed garlic	**1 cup chopped celery**

3 cups green peppers, chopped
1 28 oz. can undrained tomatoes
1 medium can red kidney beans, drained and rinsed

Place ground meat in hard plastic colander; place colander in glass bowl in microwave. Microwave on high for 3 minutes; break up. Continue cooking another 3 minutes, or until brown; stir again. In a 3-4 qt. sauce pan, heat oil and add 3/4 cup of the onions, the garlic, the celery and 1 cup of the green peppers. Saute 5-8 minutes over moderate heat, stirring occasionally, until tender. Add tomatoes, breaking them up as you stir them in. Stir in the browned meat, chili powder, basil, salt and pepper. Cover and simmer 1 hour over low heat. Uncover and simmer 40-60 minutes longer, stirring occasionally to develop flavor. Stir in the beans and cook 5 minutes longer. Garnish with remaining onions and green peppers to make it pretty. 2 cups = 1 serving.

*May make this vegetarian by adding another can of kidney beans and serving over rice or pasta.

CHICKEN OF THE DAY—your protein and your complex carbohydrate
STEAMED ASPARAGUS—part of your simple CHO
SPINACH AND APPLE SALAD—healthy munchie and the meal's added fat

BASQUE CHICKEN

1 lg. green pepper, in strips
2 med. onions, sliced and in rings
1/4 lb. thinly sliced mushrooms
2 cloves minced garlic
8 red potatoes, thinly sliced
2 chicken breasts, skinned, deboned and split lengthwise

1/2 tsp. salt (optional)
1/4 tsp. black pepper
1/4 tsp. cayenne pepper
1-1/2 cups tomato puree
1/4 cup dry white wine
1 Tbsp. water

Place vegetables in roasting pan. Place chicken pieces over vegetables; sprinkle with spices. Mix tomato puree and wine; pour into roasting pan. Bake at 375 degrees for 1 hour uncovered or until tender and browned. Pour cooking liquid with vegetables into skillet. Mix cornstarch and water; stir into skillet. Heat to boiling; cook, stirring constantly until thickened and clear. Pour sauce and vegetables over chicken and serve. This makes 4 servings; 1 piece of chicken equals your protein, two potatoes equal your complex carbohydrate, and 1 cup of sauce equals your simple carbohydrate.

STIR-FRY CHICKEN WITH CASHEWS AND SNOW PEAS

2 cloves garlic, minced
2 Tbsp. low-sodium
   soy sauce
1 Tbsp. pineapple juice
2 Tbsp. cornstarch
2 split chicken breasts,
   cut into 1-inch cubes

20 snow pea pods, sliced
1/2 cup water chestnuts,
   drained
1/2 cup chicken stock
1/2 cup unsalted raw
   cashews

Mix together garlic, soy sauce, sherry and cornstarch; marinate chicken pieces in mixture for 15 minutes. Spray wok with nonstick cooking spray, then heat with 2 tsp. peanut oil. Add chicken, stir fry for 30 seconds. Add chicken broth; stir fry until thickened. Stir in cashews; serve immediately. Wonderful over brown rice. Makes 2 servings; each gives 2-3 oz. protein, 1 simple carbohydrate and 1 added fat. The brown rice would be your complex carbohydrate.

SPINACH AND APPLE SALAD

2 Tbsp. safflower oil
1-1/2 tsp. basil
1 tsp. onion powder
1/2 tsp. salt (optional)
1/8 tsp. pepper
1/2 cup orange segments
   (optional)

3/4 cup apple juice
2 Tbsp. cider vinegar
4 cups spinach, torn in
   pieces
2 cups thinly sliced apple

Prepare dressing: In small bowl, combine oil, basil, onion powder, salt and pepper; set aside 10 minutes for flavors to blend. Stir in apple juice and vinegar. In large bowl, combine spinach, apple and oranges. Toss with 1/2 cup dressing; serve immediately. Refrigerate remaining dressing for other salads or marinade. Makes 6 healthy munchie servings and 1 added fat serving.

ITALIAN SWISS STEAK—your protein
WHOLE WHEAT NOODLES—your complex carbohydrate
STEAMED YELLOW SQUASH—part of your simple
   carbohydrate
ROMAINE LETTUCE SALAD—your healthy munchie

ITALIAN SWISS STEAK

1 lb. lean round steak*,   1/2 tsp. basil
   trimmed of fat   1/2 tsp. oregano
1/2 cup water   1 Tbsp. parsley
1 medium onion, thinly sliced 1/2 tsp. garlic powder
1 green pepper, thinly sliced salt and pepper
2 small tomatoes, cut into   to taste
   wedges
1/4 lb. mushrooms

Brown steak in nonstick skillet; add water. Place in roasting
pan with cover. Top with vegetables and water; sprinkle with
spices. Cover and bake at 350 degrees for 1-1/2 hours. Serve
over whole wheat noodles. Makes 4 servings; one serving
counts as your protein and part of your simple carbohydrate.

*May use 2 large chicken breasts, deboned, skinned and split.

EASY CHICKEN AND RICE—your protein, your complex
   carbohydrate and part of your simple carbohydrate
CAESAR'S SALAD—your healthy munchie and added fat
PEACH PIZZAZZ—more simple carbohydrate

EASY CHICKEN AND RICE
A great one-dish meal

1 whole chicken, skinned and defatted as much as possible
2 stalks celery, sliced	2 carrots, sliced
1-1/2 cups brown rice	1 Tbsp. parsley
1 cup white wine	1/4 lb. mushrooms, sliced
salt and pepper	1/2 tsp. garlic powder
1/2 onion, chopped	1/2 tsp. rosemary
1 zucchini, cubed	1/2 tsp. tarragon
1 green pepper, chopped	3 cups vegetable stock or water

Place chicken in roaster. Place all veggies, brown rice, stock, wine and seasonings around chicken. Bake covered at 350 degrees for 1-1/2 hours. You may substitute any vegetables you have: broccoli, cauliflower, okra, and so forth. When in a hurry, just top chicken with bag of frozen vegetable mix. This is the classic meal-in-one! One cup of rice equals 1 complex carbohydrate and 1 fat. Slice chicken to appropriate proportions.

CAESAR'S SALAD

4 cups washed, torn romaine lettuce
1 clove minced garlic
1-1/2 Tbsp. olive oil
1/2 tsp. dry mustard
1 tsp. Worcestershire sauce
1/8 tsp. coarse black pepper
1/8 tsp. salt (optional)
1 coddled egg*
juice of 1 lemon
1/4 cup grated Parmesan
croutons made from 2 slices whole wheat bread sprinkled
  with garlic powder, toasted till brown

Rub bottom and sides of large salad bowl with garlic; leave in bowl. Add oil, mustard, Worcestershire sauce and spices; beat together with fork. Add chilled romaine lettuce; toss well. Top with coddled egg and lemon juice; toss till lettuce is well covered. Top with Parmesan and croutons. Toss well and enjoy! Makes 6 servings. This gives a healthy munchie and an added fat.

*Coddle an egg by immersing the egg in shell in boiling water 30 seconds.

PEACH PIZZAZZ

**4 peach halves, fresh or packed in own juice,
  without sugar
3 Tbsp. Philadelphia Lite cream cheese
Cinnamon**

Place peach halves on lettuce leaves; top with 2 tsp. cheese and sprinkle with cinnamon. Makes 4 servings; each counts as part of your simple carbohydrate and a small amount of protein.

**SPAGHETTI PIE
MARINATED VEGGIES** (variety of raw veggies marinated in no-oil Italian dressing, sprinkled with Parmesan cheese)

SPAGHETTI PIE

6 oz. vermicelli or whole wheat pasta
2 tsp. olive oil
1/3 cup grated Parmesan cheese
2 egg whites, well beaten
1/2 lb. ground turkey*
1/2 cup chopped onion
1/4 cup chopped green pepper
1/2 cup shredded mozzarella cheese
1 8 oz. can stewed tomatoes
1 6 oz. can tomato paste
3/4 tsp. dried oregano
1/4 tsp. salt (optional)
1/2 tsp. garlic powder
1 cup part-skimmed ricotta cheese

Cook pasta according to package directions; drain. Stir olive oil and Parmesan cheese into hot pasta. Add egg whites, stirring well. Spoon mixture into a 10" pie plate. Use a spoon to shape the spaghetti into a pie shell. Microwave at HIGH uncovered 3 minutes or until set. Set aside.

Crumble turkey in a colander; stir in onion and green pepper. Cover with plastic wrap and microwave at HIGH 5-6 minutes, stirring every 2 minutes. Let drain well. Put into a bowl and stir in tomatoes, tomato paste and seasonings. Cover and microwave at HIGH 3-1/2 to 4 minutes, stirring once. Set aside.

Spread ricotta evenly over pie shell. Top with meat sauce. Cover with plastic wrap and microwave at HIGH 6 to 6-1/2 minutes; sprinkle with mozzarella cheese. Microwave uncovered at HIGH 30 seconds, or until cheese begins to melt.

Makes 8 servings; each equals 2 oz. protein, 1 complex and 1 simple carbohydrate.

*May substitute ground round; drain *well* after cooking.

WHAT ABOUT ANOREXIA AND BULIMIA?

The essential factor in any eating disorder is the attitude toward food and dieting. But the person with a clinical eating disorder also has a distorted image of his or her body appearance. Fat people see themselves as thinner than they really are, and even emaciated people see themselves as fat. These disorders come from internal perceptions and have nothing to do with reality. These internal messages fuel the eating relationship.

Estimates about the rate of clinical eating disorders vary from researcher to researcher. It has been estimated that as many as one out of three college women engage in some kind of binging and purging. Clinical eating disorders are not only seen in women; men are afflicted as well, and victims of the disease range from teenagers to grandparents, students to successful career people, homemakers to athletes. As in any addictive life-style patterns, one person's problems can start to control the behavior of the entire family.

Let's look at bulimia and anorexia, the two most common clinical eating disorders.

What Is Bulimia?

Bulimia is an extreme obsession with food. The word *bulimia* is derived from the Greek word *buli*, which means "animal hunger" or "to eat like an animal." (I'll never forget the first time a patient described herself as "eating like a dog.") Being bulimic is not just eating large quantities of food, and you don't have to vomit to be bulimic. Actually, vomiting is not in the definition. Instead, bulimia is related to the *way* in which food is consumed (most often in a frenzied, binging pattern) combined with some sort of "purging" (extended fasting, vomiting, use of laxatives or intense exercise). *Binging* is taking in large amounts of food in a brief period of time.

Characteristics of Bulimia

- Binging on high-calorie foods that can be taken in easily.
- Binging in secret.
- Feeling out of control with eating—unable to stop a binge once started. (To stop, the binge must be physically interrupted by a person, stomach pain, vomiting, falling asleep, and so on.)
- Feeling depressed and worthless after a binge.

196

Research shows that binging means different things to different people. Some bulimics report consuming up to forty thousand calories and taking as many as six hundred laxatives a week. Some binge every day. Some purge after any meal or snack, claiming they feel bloated and fat no matter what they eat.

Many compulsive eaters say they first started to purge in hopes of gaining relief from the guilt and bloatedness of overeating.

Although a food binge seems, and feels, out of control, it is actually all about control. You are safe and secure while binging. Your need for love is being met at a steady pace; your feelings are sedated; and you are totally in control of food. You may be out of control of every other aspect of life, but *you* buy food, you prepare it and you eat it. That makes you totally in control, not needing anyone else. When you are frightened, you most likely can't think of any way to get relief except through binging.

Anorexia: Frozen Emotions

A person with the eating illness of anorexia also has an obsession with food, but to an opposite extreme. The anorexic has an unnatural *fear* of food and is obsessed with *not* eating. As you deprive yourself of food, you sedate yourself against feelings, much as you can with binging; not eating can put you into a trancelike void of feelings. In anorexia, if you don't eat, you don't feel.

The anorexic takes the control a step further than the bulimic. By not eating he or she feels invincibly in control. By not needing food, the anorexic can also be saying that he or she doesn't need *people*. It is a desperate statement of the need for control: I want to protect myself from the need for love.

Sometimes anorexia starts with rigid dieting. Maybe some teasing about getting "chubby" or "plump" fuels a fear of food. Maybe societal pressure to be thin and glamorous is internalized in the extreme. A teenager failing an important test or try-out at school might be flooded with those I'm-out-of-control feelings. How can she gain control in one part of her life? By rigidly dieting. Criticism and concern from others often causes an anorexic's problems to worsen; as she feels rejected, she may withdraw further from people.

Getting Help

There are many groups that have formed to aid eating disorder victims and their families. These groups offer detailed information to victims and refer them to doctors and treatment centers. One such group is the National Association of Anorexia Nervosa and Associated Disorders (ANAD), Box 271, Highland Park, IL 60035.

THE TWELVE STEPS OF ALCOHOLICS ANONYMOUS

1) We admitted we were powerless over alcohol—that our lives had become unmanageable.

2) Came to believe that a Power greater than ourselves could restore us to sanity.

3) Made a decision to turn our will and our lives over to the care of God as we understood Him.

4) Made a searching and fearless moral inventory of ourselves.

5) Admitted to God, to ourselves, and to another human being the exact nature of our wrongs.

6) Were entirely ready to have God remove all these

defects of character.

7) Humbly asked Him to remove our shortcomings.

8) Made a list of all persons we had harmed and became willing to make amends to them all.

9) Made direct amends to such people wherever possible, except when to do so would injure them or others.

10) Continued to take personal inventory and when we were wrong promptly admitted it.

11) Sought through prayer and meditation to improve our conscious contact with God as we understood Him, praying only for knowledge of His will for us and the power to carry that out.

12) Having had a spiritual awakening as the result of these steps, we tried to carry this message to alcoholics and to practice these principles in all our affairs.

Reprinted with permission of Alcoholics Anonymous World Services Inc.

BIBLIOGRAPHY

Beattie, Melody. *Codependent No More*. New York: Harper & Row, 1987.

Bradshaw, John. *Healing the Shame*. Deerfield Beach, Fla.: Health Communications Inc., 1988.

Friel, John and Linda. *Adult Children: The Secrets of Dysfunctional Families*. Pompano Beach, Fla.: Health Communications Inc., 1988.

Hollis, Judi. *Fat Is a Family Affair*. Center City, Minn.: Hazelden Educational Materials, 1985.

MacDonald, Gordon. *Ordering Your Private World*. Nashville, Tenn.: Oliver-Nelson, 1985.

McFarland, Barbara and Tyeis Baker-Baumann. *Feeding the Empty Heart: Adult Children and Compulsive Eating*. Center City, Minn.: Hazelden Educational Materials, 1988.

Root, Maria P. et al. *Bulimia: A Systems Approach to Treatment*. New York: Penguin Books, 1986.

Seamands, David. *Healing for Damaged Emotions*. Wheaton, Ill.: Victor Books, 1989.

Smith, M.S. *The Challenge of Change*. Marietta, Ga.: Kennestone Hospice, 1986.

Seminars and Helpful Materials Available

Pamela M. Smith, R.D., has a private counseling practice in Orlando, Florida. She provides individual counseling, group education classes and topical seminars. She also is a nationally known speaker for business, trade and professional associations and church groups.

Other books by Pamela M. Smith, R.D., include:

Eat Well — Live Well — a combination guidebook and cookbook. This book presents "The Ten Commandments of Good Nutrition" in detail, as well as a comprehensive dining-out guide. Hundreds of recipes are included from breakfasts to light entrees to great desserts and more.

Alive and Well in the Fast Lane — a lighthearted guidebook for the whole family. "The Ten Commandments of Good Nutrition" are presented in a cartoon-like format. Includes menus for perfect breakfasts, lunches and dinners as well as meal plans for weight loss and healthy eating. Coauthored with Carolyn Coats.

Perfectly Pregnant — the expectant mother's guidebook. Latest information to nourish mother and baby properly. Included is a wonderful, proven solution for morning sickness. Tasty recipes. Coauthored with Carolyn Coats.

Come Cook With Me — a kid's cookbook. Wonderful way to teach children nutrition by having them cook. Great for picky eaters. Includes kid-proven recipes and some great manners. Featured nationally on CNN News and "The Today Show." Coauthored with Carolyn Coats.

Audio tapes are also available.

For more information on books, tapes and teaching seminars, please contact: Nutritional Counseling Services, 615 E. Princeton St., Suite 115, Orlando, FL 32803, (407) 896-1179, or Creation House, 190 N. Westmonte Drive, Altamonte Springs, FL 32714, (407)862-7565.

NOTES